MRI Physics

MRI Physics

Tech to Tech Explanations

Stephen J. Powers, B.S.R.T. (R), (CT), (MR)
South Coast Hospital Group
Fall River, MA, USA

WILEY Blackwell

This edition first published 2021
© 2021 John Wiley & Sons Ltd

The right of Stephen J. Powers to be identified as the author of this work has been asserted in accordance with law.

Registered Office(s)
John Wiley & Sons, Inc., 111 River Street, Hoboken, NJ 07030, USA
John Wiley & Sons Ltd, The Atrium, Southern Gate, Chichester, West Sussex, PO19 8SQ, UK

Editorial Office
9600 Garsington Road, Oxford, OX4 2DQ, UK

For details of our global editorial offices, customer services, and more information about Wiley products visit us at www.wiley.com.

Wiley also publishes its books in a variety of electronic formats and by print-on-demand. Some content that appears in standard print versions of this book may not be available in other formats.

Library of Congress Cataloging-in-Publication Data

Names: Powers, Stephen J. (Senior MRI technologist), author.
Title: MRI physics : tech to tech explanations / Stephen J. Powers.
Description: Hoboken, NJ : Wiley-Blackwell, [2021] | Includes index.
Identifiers: LCCN 2020026624 (print) | LCCN 2020026625 (ebook) | ISBN
    9781119615026 (paperback) | ISBN 9781119615057 (adobe pdf) | ISBN
    9781119615040 (epub)
Subjects: MESH: Magnetic Resonance Imaging | Physics
Classification: LCC RC386.6.M34 (print) | LCC RC386.6.M34 (ebook) | NLM
    WN 185 | DDC 616.07/548–dc23
LC record available at https://lccn.loc.gov/2020026624
LC ebook record available at https://lccn.loc.gov/2020026625

Cover Design: Wiley
Cover Image: Courtesy of Stephen Powers

Set in 11.5/13.5pt STIX Two Text by SPi Global, Pondicherry, India

SKY10078627_062824

If you can't explain it to a 6-year-old, you don't understand it yourself.
Albert Einstein

Contents

About the Author

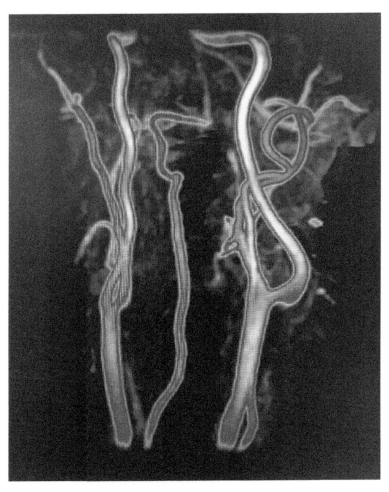

Stephen J. Powers B.S.R.T. (R), (CT), (MR)

- Received Associate Degree: Radiologic Technology, Northeastern University, Boston, Massachusetts in 1981. Bachelor of Science: Health and Social Sciences: Roger Williams University, Bristol, Rhode Island, May 1996.
- Served as MR Physics, Cross-Sectional Anatomy and Pathology Instructor: MR Certificate Program, Massasoit Community College, Brockton, Massachusetts 1999–2014.
- Clinical MR Instructor for Massachusetts College of Pharmacy 2010–2014.
- Former MR Applications Specialist: GE Health Care.
- Presently Senior Staff Technologist for Southcoast Hospital Group.
- Married with two sons and living in Southeastern Massachusetts, USA.

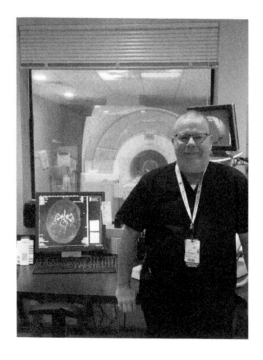

Preface

My hope for this offering is to keep it simple, one tech explaining it to another tech while drawing it on a napkin over a cup of coffee in the cafeteria.

I shall try to not use too many complicated terms, but will however have to use some. I want to keep explanations limited to what is called an "elevator speech." Some trips will go to the third floor; others will go a bit higher.

Either way, I hope to just plain say it.

Tech to Tech Explanations is not intended as an encyclopedia on MRI but hopefully a quick guide, an answer giver, a reference, or a reminder. Perhaps it will fill in some blank spots you might have, or explain something in a way that others have not.

Should you have a revelation or an "Aah ha" moment, I shall sleep well tonight. My ultimate desire is to make you a better Technologist.

Thank you for your support.

Steve

Disclaimer

I am not, nor shall I be receiving any kind of monetary endorsements, gifts, or favors from any manufacturer or vendor for mentioning their products or using vendor MR specific terminology.

Using some vendor specific terms or techniques will be inevitable in my narratives. I shall not and do not endorse any one company or vendor over another.

I shall try to be as vendor neutral as possible.

Introduction

Safety

What follows will be a generic safety offering. It is not meant to be all-encompassing or empirical.

- When in doubt, **don't.** You do not want to be "that guy."
- Magnets are always hungry. They do not make mistakes so neither can we. The magnet is always hungry. A healthy dose of paranoia has worked pretty well for me, so far.

There are three different safety considerations in MR:

1. The static magnetic field.
2. The gradient magnetic field.
3. Radiofrequency: Specific absorption rate (SAR).

The Static Magnetic Field

The static magnet field is 20 to 60 thousand or more times stronger at isocenter than the Earth's magnetic field. If something is ferrous and it gets too close, it is going for a ride. You do not want to be in between it and the scanner.

MRI Physics: Tech to Tech Explanations, First Edition. Stephen J. Powers.

> **Teaching Moment:** Magnetism is not governed by the inverse square law like x-rays are. **Magnetism has a cubic exponential relationship of attraction.** Halve the distance and there is 8 times (2^3 or $2 \times 2 \times 2$) the force of attraction. Things get drawn in very quickly. A ferrous object becomes magnetized (not just attracted but a magnet) in the presence of a strong field. Handheld and or wall-mounted ferrous detectors are now pretty much standard, as well as a series of "zone" signs as warnings. A handheld magnet is a very good idea for checking ferrous vs. non-ferrous.

We have all heard the stories and seen the pictures. From the MR point of view, there are two kinds of metals: **Ferrous vs. non-ferrous.**

- *Aluminum is non-ferrous*, i.e. it is not attracted to a magnet. It has little to no iron content.
- *Ferrous metals* include steel and alloys of iron with other metals. Manipulation of the atomic bonds between iron, carbon, and other alloys gives ferrous properties to a metal.
- *Not all stretchers, IV poles or O_2 bottles are made the same. Do not be that guy. Be paranoid.*

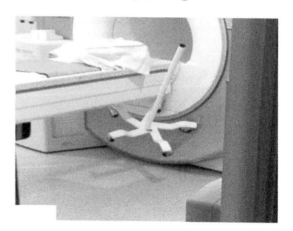

Figure I.1 Beware: Not all stretchers, IV poles, or O_2 bottles are made of non-ferrous materials.

Figure I.1 may not be an overly impressive photo of a hospital bed or respirator, but the scanner was still down for a day and a half.

The "5 Gauss line" (0.5 mT): In Figures I.2 and I.3 these are the red lines on the Gauss diagram and on the floor of the scan room.) This line is considered the "safe zone" outside of which pacemakers, defibrillators, etc. are considered safe. Each scanner has a different "5 Gauss line." Occasionally the lines are physically marked on the floor by colored tape.

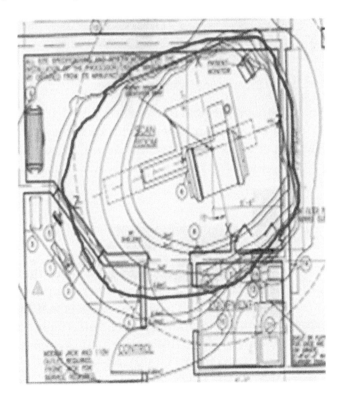

Figure I.2 The 5 Gauss line. Diagram of a scan room.

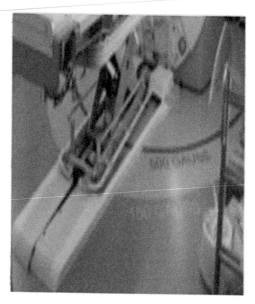

Figure I.3 The 5 Gauss line. A scan room floor.

Some mechanical medical devices and their batteries do not do well in a strong magnetic field. Parts may become magnetized or battery life may be adversely affected.

The Gradient Magnetic Field

How many patients have asked you what causes the noise? The gradients make noise as they are turned on and off. There are actually three pairs of electromagnets that superimpose themselves onto the main magnet field. They are very rapidly turned on and off, causing the banging noise. Turn it on, bang, turn it off, bang. The stronger the gradient, the louder the noise. A 1.5 T, while noisy, is usually less noisy than a 3 T.

Gradients need to work harder the stronger the static field.

What is a gradient?: A gradient is actually a hill or an incline. Have you ever seen a street or highway sign saying "Steep grade: Truckers use low gear" (Figure I.4)? It is a warning that a big downhill slope is near.

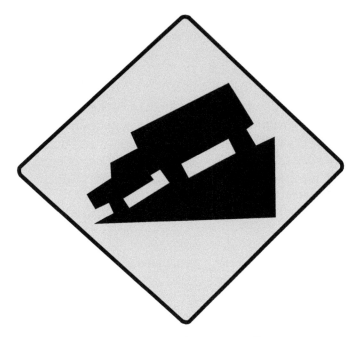

Figure I.4 Street sign warning of a steep gradient.

In MR's case, it is a magnetic hill. One side is made briefly stronger than the other. Briefly is the key word here.

Gradient Magnetic Fields and Peripheral Nerve Stimulation

Gradients are turned on and off rapidly and repeatedly, so essentially what you have are **moving magnetic fields**. The peripheral nerves in our hands and /feet are really tiny wires.

Moving magnetic fields, tiny wires, **Faraday's Law of Induction** – does this sound familiar? The oscillating magnetic fields cause tiny amounts of current to flow in the nerves, like pins and needles when you sleep on your arm.

PNS stops when the stimulus (the gradients) stops.

- You can also induce current in larger wires such as in bone growth stimulators, pacemakers, etc.
- PNS is not harmful. It is commonly caused by sequences with a lot of gradient applications. Some gradient-intense sequences include: DWI, perfusion, functional, and FSEs like those with a long ETL. FSEs are both SAR and gradient intense as well.
- On DWIs, have the phase direction in the correct direction. Many scanners now will give you a pop-up warning.
- Lower the ETL on FSEs. Each echo is caused by a 180° refocusing pulse, which also has a gradient associated with it.
- Thin slices and small FOVs cause steep gradients.

Radiofrequency and Specific Absorption Rate (SAR)

The RF energy used in MRI, circled in the electromagnetic spectrum in Figure I.5, is close to the microwave range. There will be some heating of the patient.

Some pulse sequences are more RF intense than others. Compare GRE's to Spin Echo: A GRA has only one RF pulse and it is usually less then 90°, while a Spin Echo has a 90° and a 180° RF Pulse. There is less heating during a GRE sequence. Now consider a Fast Spin Echo sequence with several 180° RF pulses. As an FYI, a Saturation band or Sat Pulse is an RF pulse.

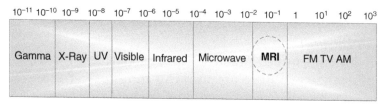

Figure I.5 The electromagnetic spectrum. Radiofrequencies used by MRI are circled.

Other considerations include:

- What body part are you scanning? Ankle or lumbar?
- What kind of coil are you using? Receive only or transmit/receive?
- Is the bore fan on? Are there lots of blankets on the patient?
- What about the patient's ability to regulate body temperature? Are they febrile? On a water mattress?

All MR rooms have what is called RF shielding or a "Faraday cage." The Faraday cage is made of copper sheets that completely cover all surfaces in the room. Like lead shielding in X-ray, its job is to keep the MR RF in, and another people's RF out.

There is a chance of RF leaks, which will of course cause artifacts in the images. Is security nearby on a walkie-talkie? Is the door not closed fully? What about the integrity of the door seal? Are those little fingers missing or bent backwards? Is there a new or different piece of equipment in the room?

Teaching Moment: Did a light bulb recently get replaced? If so, just hope it is not an LED. LEDs have a small transformer in them to convert A/C to D/C. The transformer can cause RF or data spikes (Figure I.6).

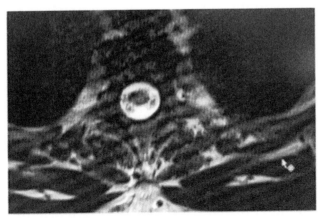

Figure I.6 Artifact caused by LED light bulb.

Your Point of View While You Are Scanning

This section is to orient you, or give you a point of view to visualize the MR physics of transverse (X/Y) and longitudinal (B_0) planes.

What a piece of paper fails to get across is that imaging modalities are 3D, whereas a piece of paper is of course 2D. So, for this book, always assume that the patient is head first and supine in the scanner.

Your point of view (POV) is not always sitting at the console looking at the sole of the patient's feet; rather you are looking down from the ceiling with the top of the magnet cut off (as if the patient is in a bath tub, the magnet being the tub).

Occasionally you will need to imagine yourself at the end of the bore looking at the patient's feet to picture the coil and transverse plane.

Try to train your brain to think in 3D. You have two eyes, so see in 3D; try to think in it as well. The Cartesian coordinate system is the three cardinal directions in MR, much as North, South, East, and West are the four cardinal directions on Earth.

- The longitudinal plane (0° and 180°) is running head to foot.
- The transverse or X/Y (90°, 270°) is right/left and actually anterior/posterior (A/P) also (Figure I.7).

Why are these "degrees" important?: They denote positions of the NMV before, during, or after the sequence as a result of the applied RF.

Note that the head coil and actually all coils are in the X/Y, also known as the transverse or 90°, 270°.

Protons pointing at the coil at the TE will be bright.

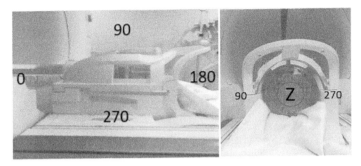

Figure I.7 The patient is head first and supine. Note that the coil is around the phantom in the X/Y, transverse or 90°/270° plane. Longitudinal, Z or B_0 is running head to feet (0–180). When you are seated at the console and looking up the bore, you are looking up the Z direction.

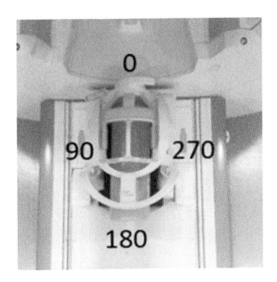

Figure I.8 The net magnetic vector (NMV) is in the longitudinal (0°/180°) prior to any RF pulses. The result of the excitation RF pulse is to move the NMV into the X/Y or transverse plane (90°/270°).

Coils relative to the patient position for longitudinal and transverse planes are shown in Figures I.7 and I.8.

Here is else to something to remember. **RF pulses are additive:** A90° pulse followed closely by a second 90° puts the NMV into the 180°.

What are you doing during an exam? **You are performing an MR experiment.**

You may have noticed in the course of scanning that every exam has a T1, T2, and some type of fat suppression. Ever wonder why? A radiologist knows what various tissues do on all weightings. They want to know if a tissue is acting like fat, fluid, or tumor. They are thinking: "Is it doing the fat, fluid, or tumor thing?" (an "if then/go to" thought process).

The T1/T2 and fat suppressed images are the "controls" of the experiment. Then you add in variables like IV contrast, a DWI or GRE to see what the region of interest (ROI) does.

How do you reason things out?

- You know that fluid is dark on T1 and bright on T2, so identifying a fluid-filled cyst is easy. If a tissue acts like fluid on all weightings, it is likely a cyst of some sort. If it does not "do the fluid or fat thing" or there is suspicion of a solid component, expect to give IV contrast to help identify different tissue or vascular characteristics. Does it do the tumor/infection thing after gadolinium?
- Another important aspect of an exam is a good clinical history. There are things the radiologist needs to know: Surgery, radiation, biopsy of the area. Those change things quite a bit. Surgery, biopsy, or radiation therapy can and will introduce blood products or tissue reactions into the lesion and change the tissue's contrast characteristics.
- Is it a new or old injury/surgery? Changes in tissue characteristics occur with duration.

All these are variables the radiologist needs to know about.

The MR Experiment in Images

The following set of images, in Figures I.9 through I.12, shows different images that are the "controls."

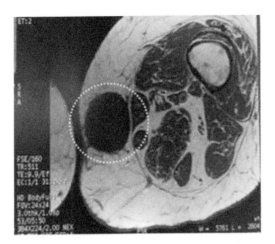

Figure I.9 T1 axial pre. A possible cyst (circled) is doing the "fluid" thing. It is **dark on a T1.**

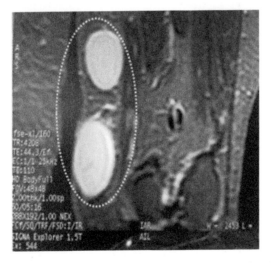

Figure I.10 **STIR Coronal.** A possible cyst (oval) doing the "fluid" thing. It is **bright on STIR.** So far, it's two for two for being a fluid-containing structure.

Gadolinium was given as the "variable" in the experiment, just before the image in Figure I.13 was taken. The radiologist uses the information taken from all the controls and the variable to decide what the region of interest is.

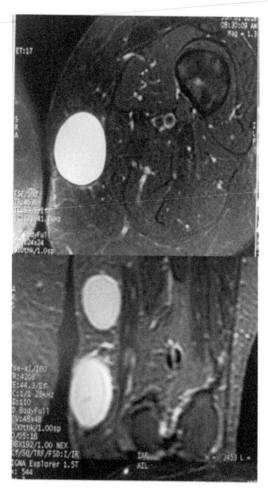

Figure I.11 Two similar contrasts: Notice that T2 FS and STIR have dark fat and bright fluid. Both T2 fat-sat (top) and the STIR (bottom) demonstrate that the ROI is not a fat-containing structure; it does not suppress. **Again, it is doing the "fluid thing," not the "fat thing," as it does not suppress like fat should.**

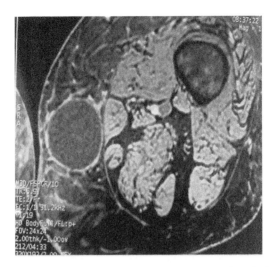

Figure I.12 T1 fat-sat pre. Pre contrast done immediately before administration of contrast. It is vital that the pre and post contrast images are scanned with the exact same TR and TE. The only difference between them should be the IV contrast.

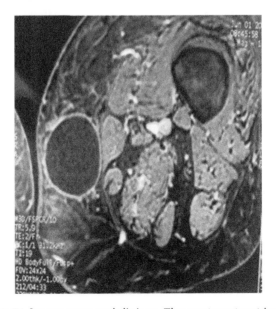

Figure I.13 T1 fat-sat post gadolinium. The post contrast image shows slight enhancement of the cyst's wall. There is no definite enhancing mass. There can be a high degree of confidence that this is a simple cyst. A mass would likely vividly enhance, and infection would have localized soft tissue inflammatory enhancement.

Notes

Acknowledgements

First, I would like to thank my wonderful wife Suzanne for all the years of patience and support during the many days, nights, weekends, holidays, call, and most recently all those many road trips while I was on the road following my passion.

The next person on my thank you list is a friend, colleague, and mentor: Annette Caballero-Saes. She has taught me a great deal on the MR Applications side of things. Her modus operandi always was "Keep it simple." That is my hope for this book. With that I say: "Thank you, Annette."

I never thought myself a teacher until I had the very fortunate opportunity to work with a fine Radiologist and friend Dr Richard Mauceri D.O. I could always ask him questions (and I had lots of them, and he would always patiently answer them. One day after a lengthy barrage of questions, I thanked him and he said to me, "Stevie, it's nice to know things that others don't so then you can show them." That statement was a life changing way of looking at things. I cannot thank you enough Dr Mauceri.

Thank you, Ashley, for your "Word" help! It was huge!

Great cover picture Rachelle! You're my favorite!

I also need to thank some very good friends, colleagues, and fellow technologists for their help in evaluating many of the chapters in this book: Manny Constantino R.T.(R)(CT) (MR), Diane Ashley R.T.(R) (MR), Susan Pius MA R.T.(R)(CT) (MR), Bernice Resnick R.T.(R)(MR)(M), and Lisa Thornhill DABR, MRSE.

1

Hardware: Magnet Types and Coils

Chapter at a Glance

Magnets

Three types of magnets are used in MRI:

- **Permanent.** These are rare to almost nonexistent today. They are made up of brick-sized magnets that, when placed in the right pattern, combine to make a magnetic field strong enough to image with. These magnets are large, heavy, and have a weak $\mathbf{B}_0$ field so signal-to-noise ratio (SNR) is at a premium. They cannot however be turned off.
- **Resistive.** These consist of a large coil of wire with a lot of electricity passing through it. The amount of electricity circulating is sufficient to make a magnetic field strong enough to image with. These are usually 0.5–0.7 T. They also generate a lot of heat from electrical resistance in the wire.

MRI Physics: Tech to Tech Explanations, First Edition. Stephen J. Powers.
© 2021 John Wiley & Sons Ltd. Published 2021 by John Wiley & Sons Ltd.

▪ *Superconducting.* These are resistive magnets but with one major difference. The magnet is cooled with liquid helium, a cryogen. The cryogen decreases electrical resistance in the wires that make up the magnet. The loss of resistance from cooling enables more current to flow so stronger magnetic fields are possible. Typical field strengths are 1–4T. Research magnets can be as strong as 7–9 T. Stronger magnetic fields also come with a larger **fringe field** compared to the lower-power fields. Think of the fringe field as being like the "Scatter Radiation" in x-radiography. The magnetic field is not solely confined to the scanner. Magnetism picks up rapidly as you get closer to the bore.

The field attraction gets stronger the closer you get to isocenter.

Teaching Moment: Magnetic force of attraction is a cubic exponential function. **Halve your distance** and the strength of the fringe field you are experiencing **goes up by a factor of 8** (2^3, or $2 \times 2 \times 2$). That is why pens, beepers, and paper clips get pulled out of your pockets and go flying into the bore at about 40 mph.

The Superconducting Magnet

The magnet coil is cooled with liquid helium. Helium is usually a gas, but when it is sufficiently compressed it becomes a liquid which is extremely cold. Liquid helium is a cryogen with a temperature of about 4° Kelvin (very close to absolute zero).

Helium does not want to be a liquid. It wants to be a gas and revert to a lower energy state. If allowed to, it will do so very rapidly. The resulting conversion back to a gas is called a **quench**. Quenches result in a high conversion ratio of about 750:1, meaning that 1 litre of liquid helium makes about 750 litres of gaseous helium. Superconducting magnets have a large vent pipe leading outside the building so that if there is a quench, the gases vent outside and do not fill the scan room.

Quenching the magnet is only done in a life-threatening situation such as when someone is pinned between a ferrous object and the magnet. Trust me, if an O_2 bottle, IV pole, or stretcher is drawn in to the magnet, you will NOT get it off. A quench will result in the scanner being down for several days.

Coils

There is a plethora of different coils. Some are general purpose; others are highly specific. General purpose or flexible coils are made by multiple manufacturers. They can be used for a shoulder on one patient, a knee on the next, then a soft tissue mass on another.

Coils for more specific use are breast, endo-rectal, or the long-lost Temporal-Mandibular Joint (TMJ) coils. If you still have TMJ coils and they still work on your system, **keep them,** they are awesome for wrists, orbits, and fingers! **Remember, a coil is a coil is a coil. But also know that coils are system specific. You cannot use a 1.5 T coil on a 3 T system and vice versa.**

Coils vary in size: small, medium, and large. If you can get it around, under, or over the area to be imaged, it will work. However, you have to choose a coil size that is appropriate to the patient size or coverage needed. **You should use the smallest coil possible for best signal to noise.** With all scan factors remaining the same, a small coil has better SNR than a large coil. Why? The smaller coil unto itself does not see more signal, **it sees less noise.** That's the signal to noise ratio. The same amount of signal with less noise results in a higher SNR.

An imaging coil is just that: loops of wire that when placed next to or around a body part form an integral part of something in MR called **Faraday's law of induction.** Faraday's law of

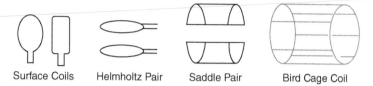

Surface Coils   Helmholtz Pair   Saddle Pair   Bird Cage Coil

Figure 1.1 The four basic coil types. Typical body parts they are used on are:

- Surface coil: spine
- Saddle coil: knee, foot/ankle
- Helmholtz: shoulder (Figure 1.2)
- Bird cage (quadrature): brain (Figure 1.3).

induction states that a moving magnet field passing through a coil of wire will induce current to flow in that wire. Current is signal, and signal is money.

Figure 1.1 shows the four basic coil types. Remember, they are no more than loops of wire. All are, in one way or another, placed around the body part being imaged. **Coils are always in the X/Y or Transverse Plane.**

Coils vary in the number of receivers that they contain. More receivers equals more signal. Remember, noise is a relative constant in the background. Protocols are built with certain coils in mind for everyday use. That is all well and good until a coil breaks or does not fit the patient. **A protocol built for an 8-channel coil is not going to look good if scanned on a 1-channel coil.** At this point you have to go to plan B. You will have to optimize the protocol to increase the SNR. The easy thing to do is add a "number of excitations" or acquisitions ("nex") or two, however, scan time will go up without affecting resolution. Consider a small increase in the field of view (FOV) (160–165), narrow the bandwidth (B/W) a bit, and drop the matrix to, say, 288 from 320. All these minor changes all gain little bits of signal, slightly less resolution, and hopefully will not affect scan time as much as just throwing nex at it.

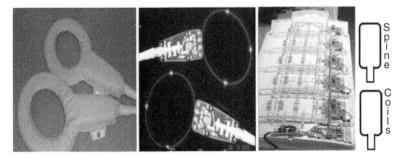

Figure 1.2 Shoulder coil or Helmholtz pair on the right. An x-ray of that same coil pair shows loops of wire with the coil electronics. On the right is a linear array spine coil with its back cover removed.

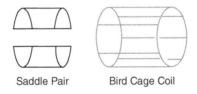

Saddle Pair   Bird Cage Coil

Figure 1.3 Typical knee and head coils.

Types of Coil

Receive Only coils

It is important to know which kind of coil you are using. Is it a receive only or a transmit/receive (T/R) coil? Why?

Images from receive only coils can have an artifact called wrap, or aliasing. This is because the scanner uses the inherent body coil (Figure 1.4) to transmit the RF. A larger area than just the coil is excited with RF and this excited tissue, even though it is not in the coil, can show up in your image and can obscure the region of interest (ROI). Excited tissue will give signal and that signal has to go somewhere. That somewhere is usually right in the ROI.

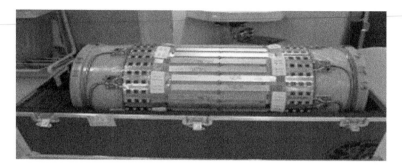

Figure 1.4 An inherent T/R body coil.

Transmit/Receive Coils

A transmit/receive coil transmits the radiofrequency (RF) to the body part, then turns off as a transmitter and becomes a receiver to acquire signal. There is little chance of wrap with these types of coil as only tissue to be imaged is in the coil and is exposed to RF. This fact decreases the whole-body Specific Absorption Rate or Ratio (SAR) as only a small area of the body is exposed to RF. This is why some implants require imaging with only T/R coils.

- Figure 1.4 shows an **inherent T/R body coil**. Note that it is a bird cage type coil (only much larger). That being said, when using a receive only coil, this body coil transmits and the surface coil receives. More of the patient is exposed to RF.
- Using the body coil to image is limited to large FOVs due to its inherent low SNR because: (i) it is a large coil, and (ii) the distance from the body part to the actual coil.

Other System Coils

Besides the inherent body coil contained in the bore there is a gradient coil (details in Chapter 13) and a shim coil(s).

The shim coil works to make the main magnetic field as homogeneous as possible. An empty bore is very homogeneous but add the patient to it and homogeneity changes. The patient is in fact the biggest contributor to magnetic field inhomogeneities. There are two shim coils: one a "hard shim," and the other an "electronic shim."

The **hard, or passive, shim** is a tube with many screw holes in it that allow small pieces of metal of various length, width, and thickness to be permanently placed into the bore to shape or "shim" the magnetic field. This is done on install.

The other shim coil is an **electronic, or active, shim**. It uses additional specialized electromagnets to correct the magnetic field. Active shims should be checked with each P.M.

Even a brand-new magnet will not meet the manufacturer's specifications. This is because the factory environment is different from the one the scanner will see when it gets to the site. At the site, there are physical differences such as the presence of other magnets, steel beams, or proximity to an elevator. After being ramped, the magnet sits for at least 24 hours to allow for "drift." The hard shim is checked, followed by an electronic shim check and adjustments if needed. The RF and coil systems are tested for quality assurance. This is just a very short list of items that are checked for manufacturing specifications.

2

The Basics

Chapter at a Glance

MRI Physics: Tech to Tech Explanations, First Edition. Stephen J. Powers.
© 2021 John Wiley & Sons Ltd. Published 2021 by John Wiley & Sons Ltd.

Need to know definitions:

- **Hydrogen (protons).** The most common molecule in the body, it acts like a small bar magnet in the main magnetic field.
- **Vector.** An entity that has a direction and a magnitude.
- **Net Magnetization Vector (NMV).** Sum of the vectors.
- **Free Induction Decay (FID).** Dephasing of protons in the X/Y plane. Also known as T2* (T2star).
- **Relaxation.** In the case of MRI, hydrogen protons returning to a lower energy state from an excited one. T2* is in the transverse plane, T1 returning to B_0.
- **Proton Density.** A tissue characteristic related to the amount of hydrogen protons in a tissue.
- **Contrast.** Signal intensity differences between tissues.
- **Signal to Noise (SNR, S/N).** The amount of signal generated compared to the background noise. It is a simple ratio.
- **B_0.** The main magnetic field.
- **B_1.** An RF field orthogonal to B_θ.

Why the Hydrogen Molecule?

The hydrogen molecule acts like a tiny bar magnet due to having a single proton (+) and electron (-). It is a small magnet or dipole. When the patient is placed into the scanner, the majority of the patient's hydrogen aligns with the scanner's north/south poles. This majority is known as a net magnetization vector or NMV. The NMV precesses or wobbles on its axis at a rate that is governed by the scanner's magnetic field strength (B_0).

Teaching Moment: At this point, the NMV is not in phase, it is just wobbling. If an RF pulse of sufficient strength or duration is applied at the precessional frequency (PF) of the NMV, the NMV will acquire phase and tip into the X/Y or transverse plane.

Why Is Hydrogen Used?

Humans are mostly H_2O, and with two hydrogen atoms and one of oxygen, the signal potential from hydrogen is higher than any other chemical in the body. We also have a good amount of fat/lipids in us as well. Fat is a long string of hydrocarbons, which can and will give off a large amount of signal. Fat and water have slightly different PFs.

- When placed into a strong external magnetic field, our protons go into a higher energy state by aligning with B_0, making it possible to produce current in the imaging coils.
- There are other chemicals in the body that can be imaged but hydrogen is the easiest and most abundant.
- How fast they "wobble" (precess) is next.

The Larmor Equation

The terms **Larmor Frequency and Precessional Frequency** are often used interchangeably. The equation for finding the Larmor frequency at any field strength is

$$Wo = \gamma B_0$$

where Wo = wobble or frequency, γ represents the gyromagnetic ratio of hydrogen at 1 Tesla, and B_0 is the magnet field strength. There are multiple ways to state the equation. The simplest and most common is $Wo = \gamma B_0$.

Very important: γ is a constant, its value never changes!
So, wobble is equal to 42.57 MHz (megahertz) times the field strength:

- Wo = 42.57 × 3T = 127.71 MHz.
- Wo = 42.57 × 1.5T = 63.85 MHz.
- Wo = 42.57 × 0.7T = 29.79 MHz.

The Net Magnetization Vector

Hydrogen is randomly aligned outside of B_0 (Figure 2.1, left), but, when in a magnetic field, the atoms align (Figure 2.1, right). The **majority** will align the correct way: opposites attract, others align north to north. Those that align opposite will negate those that align correctly. There will, however, be more that are aligned correctly than incorrectly. Those leftovers will become the **NMV** and will be the ones that produce our signal (Figure 2.2). Remember, the protons are not in-phase, just wobbling prior to RF. Phase is not achieved until the RF is applied.

The vectors that align correctly add up (net) into a larger vector: the net magnetization vector or NMV. Ultimately the NMV produces the MR signal.

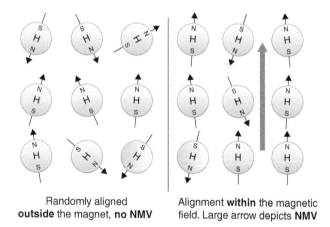

Randomly aligned
outside the magnet, **no NMV**

Alignment **within** the magnetic field. Large arrow depicts **NMV**

Figure 2.1 The net magnetization vector (NMV).

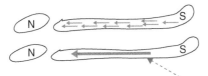

Many small vectors align making 1 large NMV

Figure 2.2 You are looking from the side of the scanner. Many small vectors align, making one large NMV. The vectors that align correctly add up (net) into a larger vector: the net magnetization vector or NMV. Ultimately the NMV produces the MR signal.

MRI is a Sequence of Events

I have heard MRI described as "knock them down and let them stand up," the "them" being protons.

With the NVM aligned with B_0 (Figure 2.3), it gets tipped into the X/Y plane by an RF excitation pulse (knocked down – Figure 2.4) and then allowed to re-align with B_0 (stand up) during a time period called the Time of Repetition (TR). The NMV is then knocked back down to the transverse plane by another 90° and allowed to relax (stand up) again. This sequence of events is repeated over and over again.

Repeatedly flipping the NMV back and forth from B_0 to the X/Y will produce current in the coil through what is called induction: Faraday's law of induction to be exact.

Faraday's law of induction may be familiar to you from high school physics or maybe Rad Tech school.

- **Faraday's Law of Induction** states that a moving magnetic field, passing through a coil of wire, produces electrical **current. That current is our signal, and signal is money in MR.**
- Now, depending on how much of a tissue's NMV is pointing at the coil when the signal is measured, a tissue will appear bright, dark, or grey. When you compare one tissue's signal next to another, that is image contrast. (You will be seeing the word **contrast** often.)
- Another factor that influences the amount of signal that is generated in the coils is the field strength of your scanner.

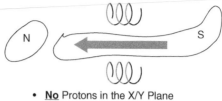

- **No** Protons in the X/Y Plane pointing at coils. No signal

Figure 2.3 The NMV aligned with the magnetic field (0/180) waiting to be excited.

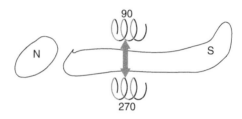

Figure 2.4 The excitation pulse moves the NMV into the transverse or X/Y plane to point at the coils.

The NMV is also larger at higher field strengths so more current (signal) is produced. All factors being the same, a 1.5T scanner produces three times the signal of a 0.5T, and a 3T produces two times that of a 1.5T.

Here is where the pictures of the coils with phantoms I showed earlier should make some sense. This is designed to get you to understand the longitudinal and transverse planes better.

The NMV (looking up the bore)

Figure 2.5 uses chopsticks to represent what happens to the NMV during a basic MRI pulse sequence. The NMV is "knocked down" into the X/Y plane by the RF at the beginning of a basic Spin Echo (SE).

Figure 2.6 uses chopsticks to represent the NMV that has been "knocked down" into the X/Y plane by the RF.

Rephasing occurs between the 180° and the Time of Echo (TE) (Figure 2.7).

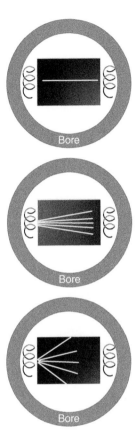

Figure 2.5 Top: The RF is "on". All protons are in phase (all together) in the X/Y or transverse plane. Middle: RF is turned off. Dephasing or T2* starts. Bottom: Over time, the "phase" that the protons had will be lost or "decay". Note that less and less of the protons (sticks) are pointed at the coil.

A quick review (Figure 2.8):

- With the patient in the scanner, protons align with the main magnet field. They are not in phase at this point.
- The 90° excitation pulse flips the NMV into the X/Y plane. Phase is produced while the RF is on.
- The RF is turned off, and de-phasing (T2* relaxation) starts.

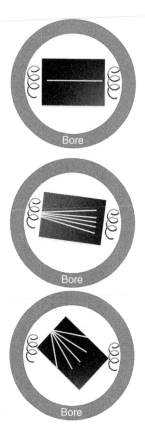

Figure 2.6 Top: The NMV while in the X/Y plane (here @90° to B_0) rotates in the transverse like a propeller. Middle: A continued de-phasing and rotation of the NMVs causes a further loss of signal. We can re-phase the NMV and get the signal back. Bottom: Note the angle between the sticks increases as de-phasing continues. After a certain amount of time we can expose the NMV to another RF pulse to bring the NMV back into phase. The second RF pulse is called a refocusing pulse or 180°.

- The 180° refocusing pulse flips protons over to start re-phasing.
- The coil is turned on to receive signal at the TE.
- Echo begins to form as the protons regain phase and are pointing in the same direction, generating an SE.

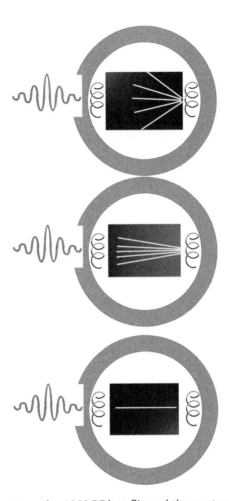

Figure 2.7 Top: Here the 180° RF has flipped the vectors to the other side and will begin to re-phase them, causing signal to start to be generated. Middle. Protons have gotten the refocusing 180° and re-phasing continues. The angle between the sticks is decreasing. The signal increases as more protons get back into phase. Bottom: Note that the amplitude of the echo is maximum as protons (NMV) come more into phase. At this point the coil is turned on to gather the signal. **The echo received from the effects of a 180° RF pulse is called a Spin Echo.**

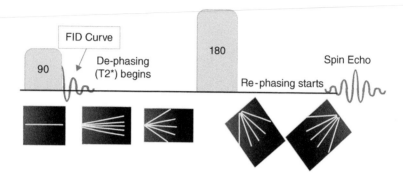

Figure 2.8 Protons diphase, then are flipped over as result of the 180°RF and begin to re-phase and will generate signal in the coil as they come back together.

Free Induction Decay (FID)

Free induction decay (FID) is the first step in the tissue relaxing. It means that the protons are **free** from the **inducing** energy of the RF, so they **decay.** Decay is the process of the vectors spreading out in the X/Y plane, also known as T2*.

The first thing to happen after an RF pulse is turned off is a very quick de-phasing or T2*. This partial "echo," as shown in Figure 2.9, is also called **FID.** T2* happens rapidly after excitation or refocusing. If you look at Figure 2.9, and you will see that the FID is really the second half of a full echo. Figure 2.10 is the next step of the SE sequence: the 180° refocusing pulse.

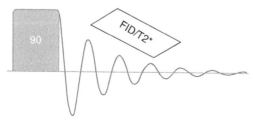

Figure 2.9 The decaying of phase (T2* or FID) after the RF pulse is shut off. A very small amount of signal is generated right after the RF is shut off. It is called an FID curve.

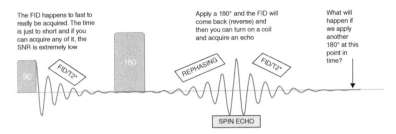

Figure 2.10 After the FID, a 180° RF causes a **Spin Echo** to form. In answer to the question: a second Spin Echo will form.

Relaxation

Relaxation is the act of something returning to a lower energy state. Given enough time, protons/NMV will reach what is called **equilibrium** (meaning they have gone to the lowest possible energy state). Outside the magnet, protons are at their lowest energy state and randomly orientated.

Putting the patient into the magnet forces protons go to a higher energy state and align either with the main magnetic field or against it. The majority align **with** B_0. **Here they are not in phase, just pointing in the same basic direction: A large NMV.** Apply an RF pulse with the correct frequency and the protons will go to a higher energy state and also acquire "phase" (all wobbling the same). Turn off the RF and they will, over time, lose phase (T2*) and go back to the next lowest energy state (T1) which is alignment with the main magnetic field (B_0). There are two relaxations: **T1 and T2.**

Both T1 and T2 relaxation are thought of as a "process." Both happen simultaneously but are independent of each other, meaning the protons are T1'ing and T2'ing at the same time. Everything wants to return to the next lowest energy state. Some go fast, others go slow.

- Relaxation is the action of protons returning to a lower energy state after the RF. RF pulses impart energy into the protons. They do not want to be at a high energy state so will go back to B_0 after the RF is turned off.

- Tissues T1 and T2 relax at different rates. We take advantage of the differences with a combination of TR and TE.

T1 relaxation is the action of the protons leaving the X/Y plane and returning into alignment with B_0. They give off their energy/ heat to the **"lattice"** and eventually reach equilibrium. T1 relaxation is sometimes referred to as **Spin-Lattice relaxation.** Tissues must T1 relax before the next excitation in order to generate maximum signal in the coil.

If another RF pulse is applied too soon, full relaxation will not be achieved, tissues will "saturate," and signal drops.

T1 and T2 Relaxation

When you turn off the RF that knocked the protons into the 90°, the NMV starts to both T2 and T1 relax.

- *T2 decay* means the protons fan out or spread out in the X/Y.
- As time passes, the protons spread out more and signal drops. **T2 is considered a decay process.**
- *T1 is a re-growth process,* meaning that the NMV is going back to B_0. It was 100% longitudinal before an RF pulse made it go to the X/Y, but when the RF is turned off, it will return to B_0 in a process called T1 relaxation.

Teaching Moment: When does relaxation happen?
Answer: When there is no RF on to keep the protons in phase and in a high energy state.

Relaxation Definitions

- The **T1** time of a tissue is the time (in ms) it takes for 63% of the NMV to **return** to B_0.
- The **T2** time of a tissue is the time it takes (in ms) for the NMV to **decay** down to 37% of its original value.

What are these numbers of 63% and 37%, and where do they come from? They are logarithmic time constants analogous to the half-life of a radionuclide.

Two Kinds of T2 Relaxation

There are actually two different kinds of T2 relaxation: True T2 or Spin-Spin interactions and T2* (T2 Star).

- *True T2 (Spin-Spin)* is when the protons (spins) bump into each other like bumper cars and knock each other out of the X/Y plane. These spins are not recovered by the 180°RF pulse. **They are not recovered until the next 90°.**
- *T2** is when the spins stay in the X/Y plane. They did not bump into each other and are recoverable by a 180° or gradient reversal. They will re-phase and generate signal at TE.

If there are two kinds of T2 relaxation, then logically there will be two different kinds of T2 curves, right? The answer is yes. I will show you two different curves. The T2 curve that is most often displayed is a best-case scenario curve. By that I mean that it is the curve you would see from an SE sequence. An SE has a 180° RF pulse correcting for the Big Three: main and local magnetic field inhomogeneities, and magnetic susceptibility. Correcting for these increases SNR and lessens artifacts. If you were to run an SE sequence, acquire multiple TEs and graph them out as data points, connecting those points would yield a T2 curve. The curve would be slightly different than that of a T2* curve but very similar. The T2*curve you could call a "real life or actual" curve where nothing is corrected for. **The T2 curve comes from the result of the 180°'s effect on the T2* curve.** Most of the time, a single T2 curve is displayed and explained. Sometimes there will be two T2 curves from different tissue. Less often is a "T2*" curve displayed and explained. Here I compare and contrast T2* and T2 relaxation curves. Figure 2.11 (top) shows both curves simultaneously. Know that there is no T2 curve without T2* and 180°s. The dotted line is a T2* curve, the dashed line **above** it a T2 relaxation curve. **Above** is a key word here, meaning it has higher signal. Both curves are all but identical.

Figure 2.11 (bottom) is a visual depiction of the effects of refocusing pulses on a T2* curve. T2* starts, and signal starts to drop. A 180° RF refocuses the protons, increasing signal by correcting for main and local magnetic field inhomogeneities as well as magnetic susceptibility differences. The resulting echo produced is called a Spin Echo. If multiple echoes were to be collected, T2* would then restart, another 180° RF gets applied, and an SE results. This continues to the end of the echo train (ET). Echo train length (ETL) shown here is nine. There will be more on ETs when I explain the "Fast or Turbo Spin Echo Sequence."

Teaching Moment: There is often confusion about the difference between T2 and T2*. A T2 weighted image or echo comes from a Spin Echo sequence: 90–180–echo. An echo coming from a gradient reversal is a T2* or GRE (Gradient Recalled Echo). The confusion is that T2*s can be T1 weighted, "T2" (bright fluid) or Proton Density (PD) weighted. The * denotation means the echo came from a gradient reversal not an RF pulse. A T1 **SP**oiled **GR**adient Echo (SPGR) post gadolinium in the liver is still technically T2*. It just shows T1 contrast. Try not to let the two T2's fool you.

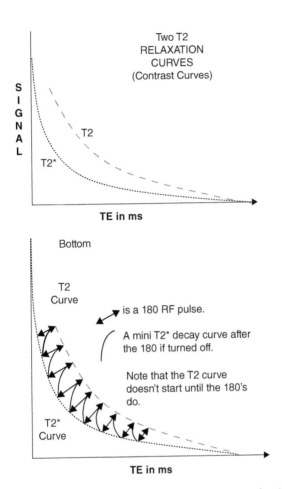

Figure 2.11 Top: The dotted T2* curve is a realistic curve having no 180°s correcting for field inhomogeneities. The dashed line is a T2 curve. It is what you get from applying 180°s to T2* decay. Note the T2 curve has a higher signal than the T2* because of the 180°s, and does not start until the first 180°. All factors being the same, SEs have higher SNR than T2* because of the effects of the 180°. Bottom: T2* decay (dotted line) always happens. The arrows represent 180°s from an echo train length (ETL). Draw a line connecting the arrowheads and you get a T2 relaxation curve. When running a Gradient Echo (GRE) sequence and you are working with the T2* curve; run an SE sequence and you are working with the T2 curve (dashed line). The graphs show that T2* happens after the 90°, a 180° is applied and an echo (a spin echo echo) is acquired, T2* starts again, another 180°, another SE echo, T2* resumes, 180° and another SE echo, T2* and so on until the end of the ET.

Proton Density

Proton density (PD) is a tissue characteristic that is sometimes termed hydrogen density. A PD image's contrast comes from differences in the amount of hydrogen protons between tissues. (FYI: There is no such thing as a PD curve.)

Tissues vary in the number of protons contained per ml (cc), for example water vs. muscle, or cerebrospinal fluid (CSF) vs. white matter. Water has more protons per ml than muscle; fat has more protons than muscle. A PD weighted image shows water or edema brighter than muscle. That is PD **contrast.**

A huge concept that is more important than anything else in MRI, or in any imaging modality, is **image contrast.**

Image Contrast

There are three prime aspects of a quality image in MRI: **contrast (CNR), signal or SNR,** and finally **resolution.** All three are needed for good Image Quality (IQ). In Figure 2.12 you see that contrast is king of the hill. Contrast is vital.

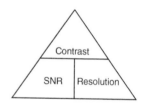

Figure 2.12 The IQ triangle.

Teaching Moment: Without good contrast between structures, all the SNR and resolution in the world does you no good.

Image Contrast Optimization

There is no equation, formula, or graph that will optimize your images. That just does not exist. Some trial and error is involved when building a protocol for the first time, followed by fine tuning.

The IQ Triangle: Contrast, SNR, Resolution

Contrast is defined as signal intensity differences between two or more tissues. Without contrast there are no images: no images = no pay check. When evaluating image quality there are three main things to consider. The most important is **Image Contrast**, next **SNR**, and finally **resolution**.

Teaching Moment: When building a sequence or protocol, get the image contrast first. Next, adjust the scan parameters to get SNR, and finally resolution (Figure 2.13).

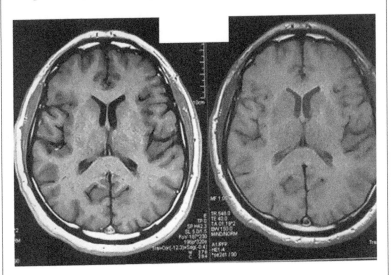

Figure 2.13 The same slice in the same patient. Left: Nice T1 contrast: good grey/white matter differentiation and dark CSF. Right: Less grey/white matter contrast, and the CSF is brighter. Recall that the combination of TR and TE is required for what makes image contrast? There are some general "limits" for the TR and TE to obtain any of the 3 image weightings. More on those limits in Chapter 3. Here, the TE makes all the difference. Left image TE is 10 ms; right is 40 ms TE. The longer TE allows some T2 contrast into the image and that is not good for T1 contrast.

Contrast to Noise Math

Contrast is signal intensity differences between tissues. As already stated, there is always noise present in MR, so, if there is not much contrast but a decent amount of noise, then the contrast to noise ratio (CNR) will be low. It is the same concept as with SNR.

Here is some "math" that may help with the CNR idea.

$$\frac{\text{Signal A} - \text{Signal B}}{\text{Noise}}$$

Breakdown: signal A minus signal B is your **contrast,** then put that over the amount of system noise, you get CNR. **You will never have to do this math, just get the concept.**

An introduction to image and the basic contrasts. Now that I have talked about T1, T2, and PD contrast, I want to take a moment to show you what they look like (or should look like) along with a short explanation of what the radiologist is looking for in those contrasts. The images in Figure 2.14 demonstrate good T1, T2, and PD contrast. **There will be much more on how these contrasts are obtained in Chapter 3.**

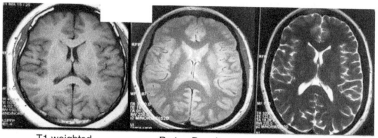

T1 weighted   Proton Density   T2 weighted

Figure 2.14 Different image contrasts demonstrated. T1: High signal intensity differences between white matter (WM) and cerebrospinal fluid (CSF); Grey matter (GM) is grey. CSF with a long T1 is dark, GM not as long so not so dark, and WM with a short T1 is bright (perhaps "White"). (WM has a high fat content in the form of myelin so has a short T1 relaxation time). PD: High signal differences between CSF and WM, WM and GM. GM and CSF have high proton densities; WM has fewer protons so is darker. T2: High signal differences between CSF and WM. CSF has a long T2, GM an intermediate T2, and WM a short T2.

Signal to Noise Ratio (SNR or S/N)

The next most important IQ concept is **signal**. Signal comes from protons that are pointing at the coil at TE. **Noise** is background hiss or static that is present in all electronic equipment. It is always there and it is **random**.

Teaching Moment: Grainy images are always an indication of low SNR (Figure 2.15). S/N is how much current is generated in the coil in the presence of noise. Hopefully there is more signal than noise.

- Grainy images just mean low SNR.
- Given the image set in Figure 2.15, the author would repeat with an extra nex or acquisition and see how they look.

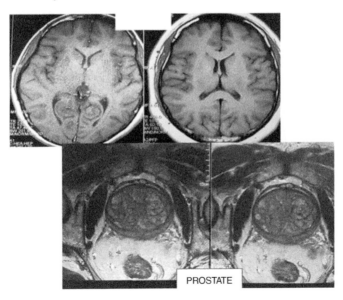

Figure 2.15 Top (brain): Left: TR 217 ms, 10 ms TE. Low SNR, good T1 contrast but grainy. Right: Good SNR and good contrast. The TR was 456 ms; the TE was also 10 ms. Bottom (prostate): Anterior coil not turned on, so low SNR. Note the general graininess of the left image.

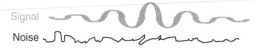

Figure 2.16 Signal and noise.

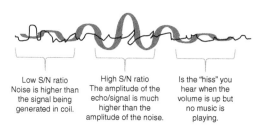

| Low S/N ratio | High S/N ratio | Is the "hiss" you |
| Noise is higher than the signal being generated in coil. | The amplitude of the echo/signal is much higher than the amplitude of the noise. | hear when the volume is up but no music is playing. |

Figure 2.17 Both sine waves are superimposed to show the idea of how much signal is generated to the amount of always present noise. This is signal to noise ratio, or SNR.

Signal (Figure 2.16) is something we create. We can create a lot or a little. Signal fades in as the protons begin to come together pointing towards the coil, reaches maximum, then fades out as they de-phase again. **Noise** (Figure 2.16) is a random, low-grade, non-useful signal inherent in all electronic equipment.

Putting signal and noise together gives you the signal to noise ratio (SNR) (Figure 2.17).

Spatial Resolution

Resolution is the ability to see or define small structures. Basically, are pixels small enough for the radiologist to see what they need to see? **The aim in MRI is to get pixels in the pathology.**

There are two kinds of resolution:

- *Spatial Resolution:* The ability to see Small Structures (see Chapter 11 for more information)
- *Temporal Resolution:* Imaging quickly over Time (see Chapter 8 for more information).

Factors affecting spatial resolution are:

- Slice Thickness.
- FOV (Field of View).
- Phase Matrix.
- Frequency Matrix.

Teaching Moment: If pixels are smaller than, or equal to a structure, that is good resolution. If they are larger, that is lower resolution (Figure 2.18).

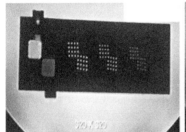 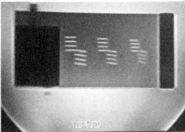

Figure 2.18 Left: High spatial resolution: pixel dimensions 320 × 320. Right: Low spatial resolution: pixel dimensions 128 × 320.

B_0 and B_1

Before I go too far, I shall explain something I have been asked many times. What is the difference between B_0 and B_1?

- B_0 is easy. It is the main magnetic field which is the core of the MR scanner. It is termed in a unit called a Tesla. The magnetic strength at the Earth's surface ranges from 25 to 65 micro-Tesla or 0.25 to 0.65 Gauss. There is no need to do the conversion math; suffice it to say that a 1 T scanner's field is 20,000 (20K) times the Earth's magnetic pull. A 7 T scanner's field is 140,000 times the Earth's magnetic field strength.

- B_1 is a secondary field that is actually an RF field. It is the RF that excites tissues in order to produce signal and is applied for the excitation and refocusing pulses.

Something not often said is that as soon as the RF is applied to the NMV aligned with B_0, it begins to gain phase coherence and flip/spin up into the X/Y plane. There is no phase prior to the RF pulse.

Teaching Moment: The Flip Angle (F/A) of a pulse sequence comes from how long the RF (B_1) is applied: A **long or short RF** pulse. The longer the RF is applied (time wise), the closer the transverse NMV gets to 90° (a higher F/A). For example, a 12° flip angle has the B_1 turned on for a shorter period of time than for a 90°. So, for a 180°, it is applied for twice as long as it was for the 90°.

Also, the amplitude/strength of RF can be changed: A short strong pulse or a longer weaker pulse. Both do the same job, but short and strong does not cost the time a long weak pulse does. If given the choice, take the short strong.

Free and Bound Protons

Not all water protons are imageable, but the vast majority are. These are the "free" ones. The others that cannot be counted on to give signal are termed "bound". This has to do with the chemical bonds that hold them. If the chemical bonds that hold them are loose enough to allow them to be "flipped" into the X/Y plane, the protons can give signal. If they are not "flippable," they will not give signal (Figure 2.19). You see them all the time and probably do not notice it.

- *Flippable:* Bone marrow, muscle, fat, synovial fluid.
- *Non-flippable:* Cortical bone, tendons, ligaments, meniscus.

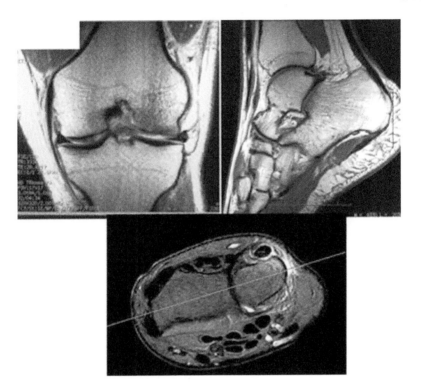

Figure 2.19 PD coronal knee, T1 sagittal ankle, and PD fat saturated wrist. Note that the cortical bone, Achilles tendon in the ankle, meniscus in the knee, and ligaments in the wrist are black because protons are bound and there is therefore no signal. Even trabecular bone is dark.

Notes

3 Image Weighting

Chapter at a Glance

This chapter covers the all-important concept of image contrast and how the combination or ratio of TR/TE is used to get good tissue contrasts or image weighting.

MRI Physics: Tech to Tech Explanations, First Edition. Stephen J. Powers.
© 2021 John Wiley & Sons Ltd. Published 2021 by John Wiley & Sons Ltd.

The concept of weighting is to have more of one thing over another. When you have a balance of two things of exactly 50/50 it is not weighted either way. An example is a half-caff coffee that is 50% caffeine and 50% decaf. It is not weighted either way. If the ratio is 70% caffeine and 30% decaf, it can be called "caffeine weighted." The same concept applies for MR images.

MR images have three primary contrasts or tissue weightings: T1, T2, and PD.

Teaching Moment: All images have some amount of all of the three weightings. There are no purely T1, T2, or PD images in everyday MR scanning.

- When an image is said to be T1 weighted, it means there are more T1 contrast characteristics than T2 or PD tissue characteristics.
- A T2 weighted image has more T2 characteristics than T1 or PD.
- Other MR images coming from advanced pulse sequences like diffusion weighted imaging (DWI) or susceptibility weighted imaging (SWI) have their own unique tissue contrast characteristics. More on those later.

Where Does Image Weighting Come From?

Image weighting or **contrast** comes primarily from different combinations of the scan parameters: TR and TE.

It is said that, in MRI, you knock the protons down and then let them stand up. TR controls who gets to stand up. If the protons get to stand up, they contribute to the signal and ultimately the image contrast.

- **TR** is the factor that controls (enhances) T1 weighting while lessening T2 and PD. Think of TR as a filter allowing only fast T1 recovering tissue to "stand up." The slow ones do not get to contribute signal to the image. A short TR means an image is more T1 than it is T2 or PD.
- **TE** controls or emphasizes T2 contrast characteristics while decreasing T1 and PD. A long TE is a characteristic of a T2 weighted image.

There is a golden rule in MR: **TR controls T1, and TE controls T2.** Here are the combinations:

- For T1 weighting: short TR, and short TE.
- For T2 weighting: long TR and long TE.
- For PD: long TR and short TE.

In the last several years, the classic PD has changed into what is called a "hybrid." It still uses a long TR (>3000 ms) but an

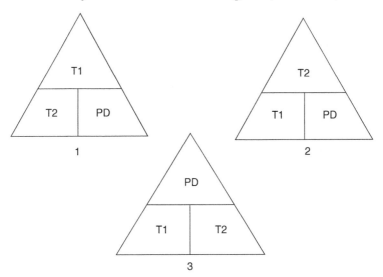

Figure 3.1 The "weighting triangle." MRI can produce only three weightings: T1, T2, and proton density (PD). The figure demonstrates that a combination of scan factors will maximize one while minimizing the other two.

intermediate TE of 30–35 ms. This is not quite PD, but the TE is not long enough to call it a T2.

This brings me to the **weighting triangle rule**: The scan parameter combination that maximizes one of the three weightings wins and goes on the top of the triangle or is "king of the hill" (Figure 3.1).

1. Short TR maximizes T1, short TE minimizes T2. **T1 wins.**
2. Long TR minimizes T1, long T2 maximizes T2. **T2 wins.**
3. Long TR minimizes T1, short TE minimizes T2. **PD wins.**

Time of Repetition (TR)

TR stands for **T**ime of **R**epetition; it is stated in milliseconds (ms).

What is a millisecond?: 1 ms is 1/1000th of a second.

There are 1000 ms in 1 second, and 60,000 ms in 1 minute. So, to put it into perspective, a TR of 500 ms = 500/1000 second or ½ a second. A TR of 4000 ms = 4 × 1000 or 4 seconds. A TR of 4 seconds (4000 ms) is the time you allowed exciting slice #1 the first time until you image it for the second time.

The 60,000 ms in a minute will come into play when we discuss scan time formulas.

Teaching Moment: All timing is in ms, whether you're talking TR, TE or TI and begins with the 90° excitation pulse.

The official definition of TR is: **the time from the first 90° RF pulse to the next 90° RF pulse that excites the same slice** (Figure 3.2). "Exciting the same slice" is key here.

TR is the time in ms to loop back to slice #1.

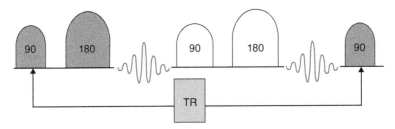

Figure 3.2 A Pulse Sequence Design (PSD). The TR is the time interval (in ms) from the first 90° to the next 90° that excites the **same** slice. Note the color of the 90° pulses. Remember that all the work needed to perform a sequence is done during each TR period.

Think of it this way: TR is a time interval that you choose to have before you repeat the slices again. It is how much time you give the scanner to do the work. Think of it as the time before you loop back around to slice #1.

> **Example:** If you set up to acquire 20 axial slices in the brain, with a TR of 600 ms, you will excite each slice, 1 through 20, once. After the first 600 ms expires, the scanner goes back to run slices 1–20 again, a second 600 ms. Then another 600 ms starts and slices 1–20 are scanned again. Do you see a pattern developing?

- Everything extra you ask the scanner to do, Sats, Flow Comp, etc., is all done during the TR.
- Extra work: Longer TRs. Longer TR: Longer scan times.
- Watch your TR in T1 land. "T1 land" is a 400–750 ms TR at 1.5 T and 600–850 ms at 3T. Be mindful to keep your TR within acceptable millisecond limits for best T1 contrast.

A notion or explanation I have heard several times during my career is that what we are doing during a TR is knocking protons down and letting them stand back up, knock them down, let them stand back up. This is repeated over and over with each TR. Depending on the chosen TR, some have time to stand back up, others do not.

Time of Echo (TE)

TE stands for **Time** of **Echo** and is also stated/measured in ms. The definition of TE is: The time from the **90° to the center of the echo**.

- TE is also sometimes referred to as 2 Tau (Figure 3.3).
- The time from the 90° pulse to the 180° pulse is 1 Tau, 180° to the echo is also 1 Tau. 1 Tau + 1 Tau = 2 Tau.
- Interpretation: **The 180° RF pulse is applied at ½ the TE.**
- The 180° is symmetrically placed between the 90° RF pulse and TE.
- Why is the 180° pulse placed at ½ the TE? If you give the protons 5 ms to de-phase, you must also give them 5 ms (the same amount of time) to re-phase or you will not get maximum SNR.

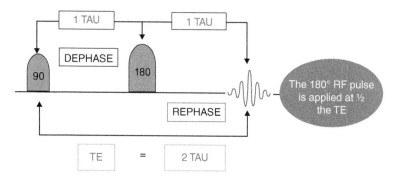

Figure 3.3 A PSD showing the TE as the time from excitation to the center of the echo. TE is sometimes called 2 Tau. The first Tau is from 90° to the 180°, and the second Tau from the 180° to signal acquisition, the TE.

Teaching Moment: A TE of 10 ms is typical for a T1 weighted image. The short TE does not allow for very much T2* relaxation to occur, so little T2 is seen in a 10 ms echo. A long TE (e.g. 100 ms) allows a lot of T2* to occur, therefore you will get it back in your echo in the form of T2 image contrast.

Teaching Moment: If TR can be thought of as a T1 filter, TE can be thought of as a T2 filter.

In other words: A long TE lets short T2 tissues both T1 and T2 and be out of the X/Y plane at the TE so they do not contribute much signal. The long T2 tissues stay in the X/Y plane pointing at the coil at TE so they are brighter. Again, **a bright tissue next to a not so bright tissue = contrast.**

The contrast seen with a long TEs is T2 contrast.

Rounding out this teaching moment: A T2 weighted image has a long TR and long TE. Also, if a tissue has a short T1, it also has a short T2. Recall the previous explanation of TR being a T1 filter; with a short TR, only short T1 relaxing tissue contrast gets through. A long TR lets both short and long T1 tissues' contrasts through. So, where will tissue contrast come from in a long TR sequence? Good question. Answer: The TE. It determines if short T1 or long T1 contrasts gets to contribute to the image contrast.

In a T2 weighted sequence, tissue with a short T1 and T2, will, during the TE, get out of the X/Y plane quicker than long T2 tissue. The long tissues hang out in the X/Y plane and have a larger NMV be pointing at the coil at TE, so will be brighter than the short T2 tissue. This equals what? Go ahead, say it: Contrast.

TE and TR

Now for the numbers. **These numbers are a general guide:**

- Short TR = 400–700 ms at 1.5 T and 600–850 ms at 3 T.
- Long TRs = 2000 ms or higher at either field strength.
- Short TEs = in the 7–10 ms range at both 1.5 and 3 T.
- Long TEs = 100–120 ms (60–70 ms with fat saturation).

Why Different TR Ranges for Different Field Strengths?

- T1 relaxation of tissues takes longer at higher field strengths because a stronger magnetic field holds the protons in place longer and stronger.
- The minimum TR at 3 T is usually 600 ms or so to decrease the chance or effects of tissue saturation.
- T2* relaxation time is hardly affected at 3 T. It does shorten a little bit but not enough to worry about.
- Keep TE times the same at 1.5 and 3 T.

Teaching Moment: Some radiologists are not too fussy about scan factors. They look at the image and if it has decent T1 contrast it is acceptable. Other radiologists are particular about the TR and TEs: Some will accept an 800 ms TR for a T1 at 1.5 T; others will not. Some may want no less than a 90 ms TE for T2 weighting; others will not. Some might want a PD with no lower than a 3500 ms TR.

Teaching Moment: The reason for such a long TR on PD images is to minimize T1 contrast contribution to the PD weighting.

How Does TR Control T1?

In order to be able to provide any signal, protons need to be flipped into the transverse plane (knock them down) and allowed enough time to return to B_0 (let them stand up). Some tissues (fatty tissues, gadolinium, and proteins) relax quickly, while other tissues (water/edema, CSF, or urine) return slowly.

Teaching Moment: Another way to think of using shorts and longs is this: If you image quickly (use short TR and TEs) you will see the short T1 relaxing tissues. Use long TRs and TEs and you will see long T1 tissues. If you remember **Fa**t is **Fa**st to T1 and T2, and water is slow to T1 and T2, you should be OK.

- When you use a short TR, long T1 relaxing tissues like fluids are not given time to return to B_0 so they generate little to no signal. You knocked them down and they did not get to stand up. The short T1 relaxing tissues did have enough time to relax (stand up) so did generate signal (bright: fat, gadolinium, and proteins).
- A short TR does not let the long T1 relaxing tissues go back to B_0. You knocked them down, but the short TR did not give them enough time to stand back up.

Teaching Moment: Recall that a short TR filters out the long T1 tissue. Short TRs will not let long T1 tissues T1 relax sufficiently. When they do not get enough time to relax, they saturate from multiple quick 90° RF pulses. The same can be said for long TEs. They let a short T2 relaxing tissues NMV get mostly out of the X/Y plane leaving the long T2 relaxing tissue behind to generate signal.

What Does TR Affect?

Besides T1 contrast, TR affects a couple of other aspects in MRI. First it affects **the patient's RF exposure (specific absorption rate – SAR) and it affects the number of slices you can acquire (the coverage).**

What is happening during the TR is that after imaging slice 1 with a 90° and 180°, the scanner moves on to slice 2, which will also get a 90° and 180°. While slice 2 is being imaged, slice 1 begins to **T1 relax, which is also cooling off.**

- If TR is short, not much cooling happens but T1 contrast is maximized (dotted arrow in Figure 3.4).
- If TR is long, then the T1 contrast decreases (circled). The distance between the two lines decreases (top right) but the slice gets to cool off quite a bit.

A quick mention about the graph in Figure 3.4:

- Each line represents a different tissue. The closer the lines are, the less T1 contrast between the tissues.
- As TR increases, there is more time for tissues to T1 relax and start to "blend" or look the same: Low T1 contrast.
- Increased TR = more tissue cooling.

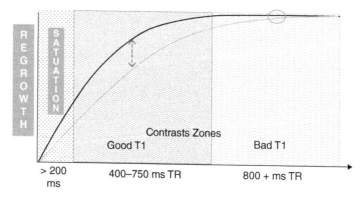

Figure 3.4 T1 contrast curve diagram.

Interpreting the T1 Relaxation Curve

Both curves in Figure 3.4 start at zero and grow over time. This growth represents increasing SNR and increasing T1 contrast to a point. The T1 contrast starts to decrease to the right, which represents a long TR. Starting with zero T1 contrast and signal, the two tissues relax at different rates. Eventually the gap between them grows over time (↑ T1 contrast) but goes back to zero over time from a long TR. Here the upper line of the curve represents a bright signal intensity tissue while the lower line is darker in signal.

Look again at Figure 3.4. An image taken too early (very short TR, 200 ms or less) will suffer from poor SNR due to **Tissue Saturation** and look grainy. Grainy images always indicate low SNR.

- An image taken at the TR of the *dotted arrow* will demonstrate good T1 contrast and good SNR.
- An image taken at the TR *circle* will demonstrate poor T1 contrast but high SNR.
- Note the different T1 contrast zones. Early =↓ SNR; middle = good T1 and SNR; late = bad T1 contrast.

Time of Repetition: Effects of the TR

TR affects the number of slices or coverage

It takes a certain amount of time to excite (90°) and refocus (180°) then acquire an echo for each slice. If the TE is 10 ms and you need 20 slices, that is 200 ms ($20 \times 10 = 200$). After you acquire the echo, you are done with that particular slice until the next TR. We know that the shorter the TR the better the T1 contrast, but use too short a TR and SNR will suffer at any field strength. We would all like to scan very quickly but, if we use the above math, using a 200 ms TR is just too short and IQ will suffer. You will get tissue saturation with a TR of 200 ms at 1.5 T. That is why a TR of 400 ms is usually the lower limit for TR. From the above math, you really only need 200 ms for the 20 slices but, to avoid saturation and improve IQ, you scan with a 400 ms TR. If you are thinking that half your scan time is spent doing nothing except giving tissue time to T1 relax, you are correct. Nothing is free in MR. Remember, saturation comes from not giving tissues enough time to T1 relax (stand up). Use too short a TR and you are hitting them with another RF pulse before they are ready.

Teaching Moment: Protons need to get knocked down and be allowed to stand up (T1 relax) or they cannot give signal. Low signal is seen as a grainy set of images.

The effects of TR on image contrast (at 1.5 T) can be seen in Figures 3.5 and 3.6.

Teaching Moment: White matter has a higher fat content than grey matter from its myelin. Myelin is mostly composed of lipids. White matter will do the "fat thing" as described in the section: "How Does TR Control T1?"

TE: The T1 and T2 of it

- The Golden Rule: TR controls T1; TE controls T2. Always!
- TEs at 1.5 or 3 T are really the same, meaning that a short TE at 1.5 is also considered a short TE at 3 T.
- For T1 contrast, a 7–10 ms TE is typical.
- For T2 contrast, a 90–120 ms TE is typical.

Short TEs do not make images more T1, they just make them less T2.

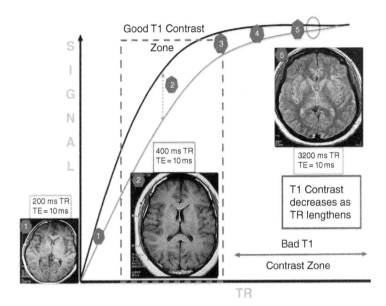

Figure 3.5 Image 1. There is low SNR due to saturation. The image has good T1 contrast but is grainy. Acquired in "**saturation zone**." Image 2. There is good SNR and T1 contrast; CSF is dark and there is good grey/white matter differentiation. Acquired in the "**good T1 contrast zone**" (400–750 ms TR at 1.5 T and 600–850 TR at 3 T). Image 5. Heavy PD contrast with darkening of white matter and brightening of grey matter. Image acquired in the "**bad T1 contrast zone**." As in Goldilocks and the Three Bears, you do not want a TR that is too short, or to long, you want it "just right."

Here is a Trick: On T2 fat-sats, try a shorter TE (e.g. 65–75 ms). You do not need a long TE on T2 fat-sat. For T2 contrast, the long TE lets fat do most of its T1 and T2 relaxing and be mostly out of the X/Y plane at TE. **With fat saturation, there is no fat to be in the way,** so if you use TEs >100 ms on fat saturation sequences, SNR will dramatically drop.

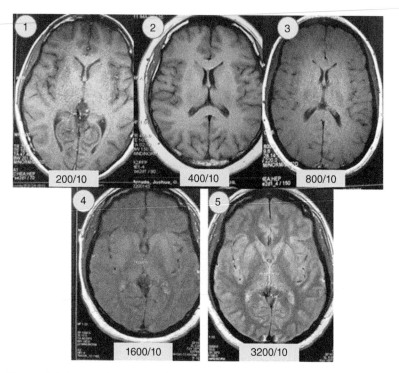

Figure 3.6 Larger images for better visualization, taken at five different TRs along the T1 curve Images 1 and 2, see legend for Figure 3.5. Image 3. There is little T1 contrast; CSF is still dark. **On the edge.** Image 4 – PD. There is a little T1 contrast (TR not long enough), brightening of CSF, and good SNR. A long TR will decrease T1 contrast, which is what a Radiologists wants on PDs. Image 5, see legend for Figure 3.5.

> **Teaching Moment: Consider all fat suppressed sequences signal starved.** Big hits to SNR on fat-sats will not end well IQ wise.

Interpreting the T2 Relaxation Curve

The two curves in Figure 3.7 start at high SNR which decreases over time. The drop means **fewer protons are pointing at the coil in the X/Y plane at any given TE.**

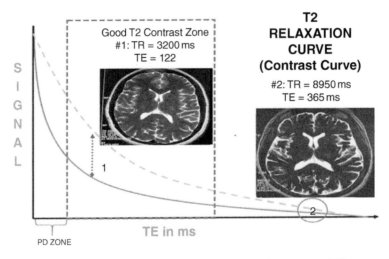

Figure 3.7 Typical T2 curves representing signal intensity difference. The dashed line is a slower but brighter tissue compared to the solid line which is a faster T2 and darker when compared to the dashed line. #1 is taken in the T2 "Goldilocks" zone. White matter is the solid line while CSF is the dashed line. #2 is taken way out with a very long TR and TE. The only thing giving signal is CSF.

- The space between them starts at zero, but as the two tissues T2 relax at different rates, the gap between them grows over time (increasing T2 contrast) and eventually goes to 0, meaning little to no signal and of course no contrast.

- Position #1 on the graph depicts good T2 contrast and good SNR. **Image contrast at 3200 TR and 122 ms TE.**

- At position #2 the curves are very close, meaning the T2 contrast in the brain is non-existent. **Scan factors: 8950 TR and 365 ms TE.** Fluid is very bright while nothing much else is. (This looks more like a Magnetic Resonance Cholangiopancreatography (MRCP) image).

- Early in the T2 curve is the PD zone (long TR/ short TE).

Teaching Moment: Which is More Important, T1 or T2 Contrast?: Each has its own usefulness, but, in general, T1 is used for anatomy and post gadolinium imaging and T2 shows pathology. T2s can be termed "pathology weighted." Given the choice, a radiologist would want T2 weighted images because fluids are bright on T2. The body's reaction to an insult – trauma, infection, surgery, or tumor – is to force fluids there. That is why a T2 image is the weighting of choice.

If you have only one contrast to hand in, make it a T2.

Effects of TE on Image Contrast

See Figure 3.8.

Teaching Moment: White matter gets darker at long TEs. It has a shorter T1 due to a higher lipid content while grey matter gets brighter due to a higher water content. White matter is doing the "fat" thing, and grey matter is doing the "water" thing.

What Do the Lines on the Curves Really Mean Anyway?

The lines, and there are usually two of them for comparison, represent different relaxation rates between the tissues. What the lines are telling you, besides one being faster and other one slower, is the contrast between them. One tissue will be bright, the other not as bright on the image, and that is **contrast.** The more "space" between them, the higher the contrast (Figure 3.9).

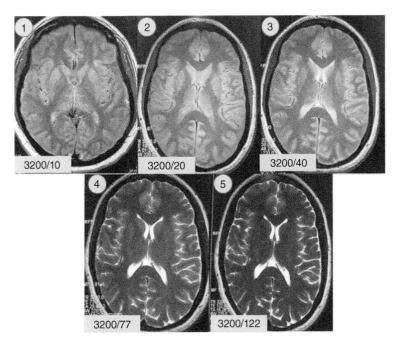

Figure 3.8 Image 1 – PD. CSF is not so bright. Some white matter (WM)/grey matter (GM) differentiation from the long TR and short TE. Image 2: 20 ms TE. CSF a bit brighter, a little more GM/WM differentiation. Image 3: 40 ms TE. CSF is even brighter from longer TE. Better GM/WM differences. Image 4: 80 ms TE. Just at the T2 contrast zone. Differences in GM/WM differences are better seen, again due to the long TR and TE. Image 5: 120 ms TE. Well into T2 contrast zone with bright CSF and good GM/WM contrast.

In a T1 curve, the top line is faster and brighter than the bottom line which is slower and therefore darker. In a T2 curve, the top line is slower and brighter.

The tissues represented by the top lines will be the brighter of the two tissues on an image. On the T1 curve: fat is on top, CSF on the bottom. On the T2 curve: CSF is on top, fat on the bottom. Note how the T2 curve is labelled a "contrast curve." The same can be said for T1 curves. The space between the lines is the difference in signal intensity, and that equals **contrast.**

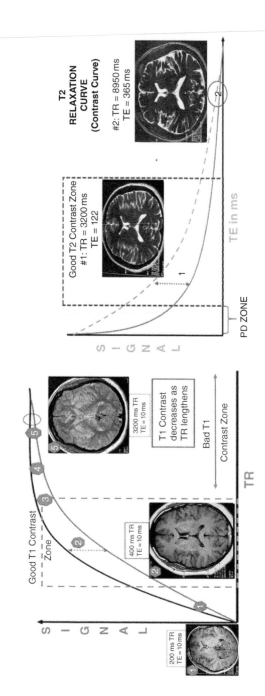

Figure 3.9 Figures 3.5 and 3.7 side by side for comparison.

One Last Weighting Triangle

So far, I have only talked about maximizing one of the three image contrasts. What happens if you maximize **both** T1 and T2 contrasts with a short TR (477 ms) and long TE (104 ms)? It will look something like Figure 3.10.

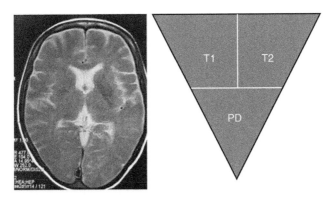

Figure 3.10 The short TR maximizes T1 so fat, gadolinium, and proteins will be bright, while a long TE will maximize T2 contrast, so CSF is also bright. GM/WM differences are poor.

Teaching Moment: Both grey and white matter are there in Figure 3.10, and right next to each other. Why do you not see any contrast between them? Answer: If two tissues are equally bright, or dark, there is no contrast between them.

- Looking at it quickly, it is easy to call the image T2 weighted.
- Submit this set of images and you will get a phone call from the radiologist, who will either be confused or annoyed or both.
- Hopefully you will not hand in images like this, but just in case you wondered what the combination looks like.

(I do not know how to draw a contrast graph for this image contrast.)

T1 and T2 Contrast Review

This chapter has been about tissue contrast. There have been definitions of it, relaxation and decay curves of it, and some basic scan parameters for it. The displayed images, however, were rather small. This short review is done with larger and better labelled images of T1 and T2 contrast. Brain images are used as that is where good T1 and T2 contrast is very important.

- T1 weighted images display short (fast) T1 relaxing as bright, with long or slow T1 relaxing tissues as darker.
- T2 weighted images show long T2 relaxing tissues as bright, with short or fast T2 relaxing tissues being a bit darker.

The two images in Figure 3.11 are from the same patient and the same slice location. On the left is a T1 showing excellent grey/white matter differentiation. White matter, with its high myelin content, acts much like fat. It is bright on a T1 because of its short T1 relaxation time. The grey matter on the other hand, with a high water content, is darker on T1 because water has a long T1 relaxation time. On a short TR, short TE image, when you see bright fat and dark water this equals T1 contrast.

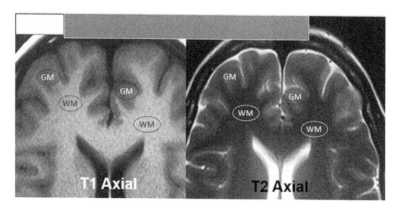

Figure 3.11 White Matter (WM)/Grey Matter (GM) differentiation.

The image on the right is T2 weighted. White matter, again a mostly fatty tissue, is darkening due to the long TR and TE. Fat has short T1 and short T2 relaxation time. The grey matter, a mostly water containing tissue, is brighter due to the long TR and TE. Water has long T1 and T2 relaxation times. It is doing the "water thing."

Earlier in this book, I said that if you image fast (by using a short TR and TE), you will see short (fast) T1 tissues brighter than long (slow) T1 tissues, and if you image slow (by using a long TR and TE) then you will see long (slow) T2 relaxing tissues brighter than the short T2 relaxing tissues.

This all leads back to **image contrast.** Image contrast is seeing signal intensity differences between tissues.

Notes

4

Introduction to the Basic Pulse Sequences

Chapter at a Glance

What is a Pulse Sequence?

- A pulse sequence is a **rigidly** timed series or sequence of events including RF pulses, gradient pulses, and echo sampling.
- There are no variations in the timing of these events.

All pulse sequences start off with an excitation RF pulse and a slice select gradient applied simultaneously. After that, depending on which kind of sequence is being run, there is a refocusing mechanism of either an RF pulse or a magnetic

MRI Physics: Tech to Tech Explanations, First Edition. Stephen J. Powers.
© 2021 John Wiley & Sons Ltd. Published 2021 by John Wiley & Sons Ltd.

field gradient. This refocusing mechanism causes an echo to form. The echo is collected by the coil, digitized, and stored in k-space.

That is the simplest description of an MR pulse sequence.

Did you know that there are only two kinds of pulse sequences: **spin echo** and **gradient echo**? All the other pulse sequences – DWI, STIR, FLAIR, SPGR, and the like – are variations of either a GRE or SE.

I am going to start off with the Spin Echo, SE, or CSE (Conventional Spin Echo). It is the simplest sequence to understand and to dissect its pulse sequence diagram (PSD).

Spin Echo (SE)

When you hear the term spin echo, automatically think **a 90° RF pulse, a 180° RF pulse, then an echo.**

It is called spin echo because the 180° RF pulse "spins" the protons in order to create an echo, hence the name "spin echo." Of all the pulse sequences, the SE is the Gold Standard for good SNR and being less sensitive to artifacts.

Spin echo is the backbone of MRI. Its structure again is: a 90° RF **slice excitation** pulse followed by a 180° RF **slice refocusing** pulse. An echo (a spin echo) results from the effects of the 180° RF pulse (Figure 4.1).

Note that in Figure 4.1 the 180° RF pulse is "taller," meaning it has a higher amplitude or has more RF in it than the 90° RF pulse. This fact is significant when we start talking about and comparing GRE sequences, especially when it comes to SAR levels.

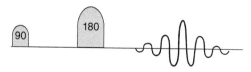

Figure 4.1 A spin echo line diagram in its simplest form. The classic characteristic of an SE pulse sequence is a 90° to 180° RF complex followed by echo formation.

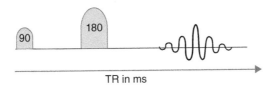

Figure 4.2 A basic PSD, as seen in Figure 4.1. TR is displayed as beginning at the 90° and **counts up or increases** going right.

How to Read a Line Diagram or PSD

PSD is short for pulse sequence design.

Figure 4.2 is a repeat of Figure 4.1 with a minor difference; it shows that in both an SE and GRE sequence, the TR starts at the 90° RF pulse. When I start talking about the different RF pulse applications, and especially the magnetic field gradients, the following explanations will be applicable.

- Items above the line are positive (+), and those below the line are negative (-).
- Time runs from left to right.
- Soon additional items will begin to appear such as the SSG, PEG, FEG, and ADC, and the PSDs will get more complicated.
- SSG = slice select gradient.
- PEG = phase encoding gradient.
- FEG = frequency encoding gradient.
- ADC = analog to digital converter.

Conventional Spin Echo (CSE)

The 90° RF pulse excites the slice to be imaged, then a 180° RF pulse refocuses the de-phasing (T2*) that occurs after the 90° RF is turned off. Protons will re-phase and point at the coil, creating an echo for that slice. Recall I stated earlier that the CSE sequence is rather artifact insensitive? Not immune to them but insensitive. This comes from the effects of the 180°

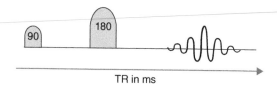

Figure 4.3 The same basic PSD as in Figures 4.1 and 4.2. Note the position of the 180°. It is at half (½) the TE. Its job is to correct for or clean up the effects of the Big Three. These are local and main magnetic field inhomogeneities, and magnetic susceptibility.

RF pulse. Besides refocusing and creating an echo, it cleans up for or corrects for the effects of three different things: **local and main magnetic field inhomogeneities, and magnetic susceptibility** (Figure 4.3).

"The Big Three" are listed here:

1. **Local magnetic field inhomogeneities** are just that, small localized impurities in the magnetic field caused by several things: surgical clips, air, or perhaps blood in the brain from trauma, surgery, tumor, or simply different tissues right next to each other. See Figure 4.4.

2. **Main magnetic field inhomogeneities** are larger inconsistencies of the main magnetic field. Causes could be service-related issues such as the field shim drifting or metallic foreign objects being drawn into the bore. The patient is actually a big cause of both kinds of magnetic field inhomogeneities.

3. **Magnetic susceptibility.** Some tissues cannot be magnetized while others can. Air, for example, cannot while muscle, liver, and CSF can. The tissues that cannot be magnetized will warp the magnetic field ever so slightly and affect the tissues around them. This causes a "bloom" or signal loss at their interface. You see this with GRE sequences in the brain where the air sinuses cause a signal loss that creeps into the brain.

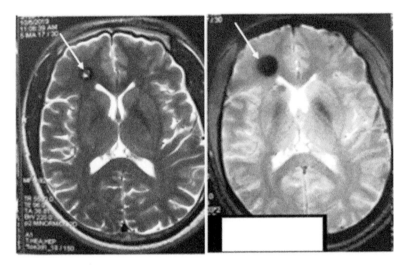

Figure 4.4 Susceptibility is demonstrated in the right frontal area (arrows) on this SE (left), and on a GRE (T2*) (right) from a small area of hemorrhage. Same patient and same slice.

Teaching Moment: The patient is the biggest source/cause of field inhomogeneities and susceptibilities due to bone, air, metal, and any number of other things.

Gradient Echo/Gradient Recalled Echo (GRE)

GREs are called T2* (T2 star).

The basic GRE PSD starts off just like an SE with a slice select excitation pulse, **which is usually something less than 90°** but can be as much as 90°. After the excitation pulse, a **gradient** is applied to refocus the de-phasing, not a 180° RF pulse. Note that while a gradient cannot excite a slice, it can be used to refocus it. The echo resulting from this **gradient** application is called a "**gradient echo**" or gradient recalled echo (GRE), hence the name of the sequence.

■ GREs, which have no 180° RF refocusing pulse, are sensitive to that which the 180° cleans up for, that being: **local** and **main** magnetic field inhomogeneities and **magnetic susceptibilities** (the Big Three).

■ This is why you routinely run a GRE in the brain (usually axials) in case there is any chance for hemorrhage. **In actuality, you are looking for a susceptibility artifact.**

■ Blood will cause this artifact. Blood has hemoglobin, hemoglobin contains iron, and iron causes small areas of susceptibility. The radiologist and especially the referring MD really want to know if there is blood in the brain. It is not unusual to see petechial hemorrhage in a tumor or post trauma. Blood in the brain changes the course of treatment (Figure 4.4).

There will be explanations of GRE contrast weightings and scan parameters in Chapter 7.

Line Diagram Anatomy

■ Spin echo (Figure 4.5).
■ Gradient echo/gradient recalled echo (Figure 4.6).

GRE line diagram anatomy is shown in Figure 4.7.

Teaching Moment: Both sequences are remarkably similar. The **major** difference is the lack of a 180° RF pulse in a GRE.

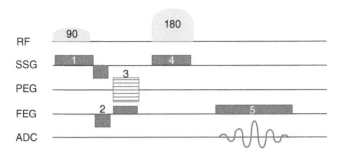

Figure 4.5 The CSE sequence. 1. A 90° **RF** pulse and a slice select gradient **(SSG)** are applied simultaneously. (just like in GRE). 2. Immediately after that, the read gradient **(FEG)** and a negative SSG are applied to re-phase the protons that were affected by the first **SSG**. 3. The phase encoding gradient **(PEG)** is applied. The phase gradient assigns which line of *k*-space the echo will go into. Then wait (half the TE) for de-phasing. (The 180° is described as being "symmetrically" placed between the 90° RF and TE, i.e. at half the TE.) 4. At half the TE the SSG and a 180° pulse are applied to re-select the slice and refocus those protons. 5. At the TE, the frequency or read gradient is applied to sample the echo (just like in GRE, Figure 4.6).

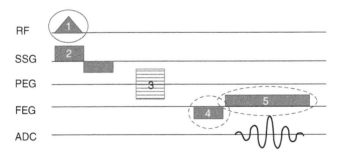

Figure 4.6 A simplified example of a gradient echo PSD.
  ▧ The slice select RF excitation pulse is circled.
  ▧ After time for de-phasing, another set of gradients are applied (dashed circles 4 and 5), causing an echo to form.
1 **RF**: Slice excitation pulse; 2 **SSG**: Slice select gradient; 3 **PEG**: Phase encode gradient; 4 and 5 **FEG**: Frequency encoding gradient. **ADC**: Analog to digital converter (receiver coil).

  Do not worry about knowing the what's, when's and why's for each of these sequence applications right now, just get the **"gradient echo"** concept of the diagram. The echo formed from the gradient reversal/refocusing will be affected by the effects of the Big Three.

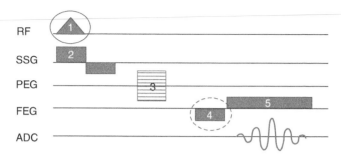

Figure 4.7 The GRE sequence. 1. The slice select gradient (SSG) and an RF pulse are applied simultaneously (just like in SE). 2. A negative SSG is applied to re-phase the protons that were affected (de-phased) by the application of the SSG. 3. The phase encoding gradient (PEG) tells the scanner which line of *k*-space the future echo should go into. Then we wait, half the TE actually, for de-phasing to happen. 4. At half the TE a negative frequency gradient is applied (4) followed by a positive (5) to refocus the protons. 5. At TE, the frequency or read (FEG) is applied to sample the echo by the ADC (just like in SE, Figure 4.6).

Line Diagram Anatomy Review: Both SE and GRE sequences start off with simultaneous RF pulses and an SSG. Phase encoding happens next and the sequence ends with simultaneous frequency encoding or readout gradient application to read the echo at TE.

Teaching Moment: To remember the order of the gradients, think **SPF** (slice, phase, frequency), just like **S**unscreen **P**rotection **F**actor seen on bottles of sun tan lotion (e.g. SPF 30).

Remember, this sequence of events happens for each slice, over and over again, for as many lines of phase as you have in your phase matrix.

The Ernst Angle

The **Ernst angle** is a flip angle that will produce maximum signal and T1 contrast for a given TR. The Ernst angle is not often used or mentioned in MRI. It is more often used at 3 T for better T1 contrast. It is also known as "T1-MEMP". This only applies to an **SE sequence**, not turbo spin echo. The drawback can be long scan times. The flip angle in a conventional SE is always assumed to be 90°. There is, however, a connection between flip angle and TR for good T1 contrast.

In a GRE or SE sequence, increasing the flip angle will increase SNR and T1 contrast. Higher flip angles put more protons into the X/Y plane so signal increases, and vice versa. Tissues have their own T1 relaxation times, so if the flip angle is increased with a constant TR/TE, SNR increases to a point, then starts to decrease. The point where SNR starts to drop is called the Ernst angle. This means that the tissue has sufficient time to T1 relax during the TR as the flip angle increases until, at a certain flip angle, the TR does not give enough time for the tissue to T1 relax. **SNR starts to drop as tissues begin to saturate past the Ernst angle.**

Figure 4.8 shows that the dotted tissue begins to saturate at about a 50° F/A, whereas the dashed tissue starts to saturate at about 40°. **TR/TE are constant.**

What are the benefits of using the Ernst angle?

- It can help to get better T1 contrast at 3 T.
- Flip angles can be used to decrease the SAR, especially at 3 T.

What does it look like on an image? In Figure 4.9 F/A increases, from 12° at top left, to 45° top right, and finally to 90° in the bottom image. Note the signal drop with increasing F/A.

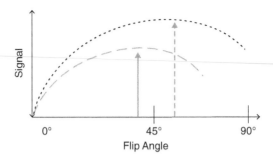

Figure 4.8 A T1 curve of two different tissues. This diagram shows the signal differences of two tissues with different flip angles for a given TR. All tissues will give more signal as the flip angle increases, but only to a certain point. At some point, the tissue cannot T1 relax fully during the stated TR and will begin to saturate. So, the dotted tissue's Ernst angle is, say, 50° at a given TR, whereas the dashed tissue drops in signal at, say, 40° for the same TR. The point where signal begins to drop is known as the Ernst angle.

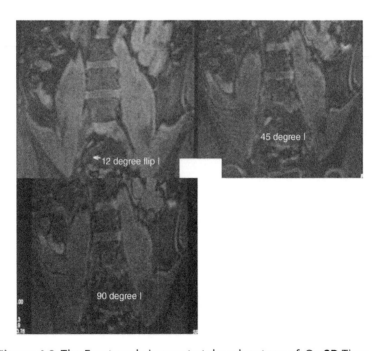

Figure 4.9 The Ernst angle is easy to take advantage of. On **2D** Time of Flight images (TOFs), simply increase your F/A into the 75–85° range and signal from background tissue drops, making maximum intensity projections (MIPs) easier. On **3D** TOF Contrast Enhanced Magnetic Resonance Angiography (CE-MRA), it works the same way. Applying a higher F/A is like a poor man's fat-sat. You get a similar background suppression effect without the time penalty of a fat-sat RF pulse.

Notes

5 Multi Echo Spin Echo Sequence

Chapter at a Glance

MRI Physics: Tech to Tech Explanations, First Edition. Stephen J. Powers.
© 2021 John Wiley & Sons Ltd. Published 2021 by John Wiley & Sons Ltd.

The multi echo spin echo sequence is also known as fast spin echo (FSE) or turbo spin echo (TSE).

The multi echo (FSE/TSE) sequence starts off with the conventional SE 90°/180° RF pattern, but adds multiple 180°RF pulses, each producing an echo. Each echo fills another line in *k*-space, thus decreasing scan time. In Figure 5.1, there are two 180°s so two echoes per TR per slice This would halve the scan time. Add three 180°s and scan time is cut to a third; add four 180°s and it is cut to a fourth. See a pattern? The multiple echoes per slice per TR is called an echo train (ET).

With multiple echoes being produced during a TR, it means that the multiple contrasts must be managed. This is done by adjusting several scan parameters. At this point, I need to introduce *k*-space: What it is and how it works.

Introduction to *k*-Space

k-**Space** is not such a dark and scary place. It is actually an easy concept. First, what is it? **It is a place to put your stuff.** That stuff is your raw data or echoes. *k*-Spaces do not truly "exist." You cannot touch them. They are arbitrary, temporary entities that live in the memory of the scanner's computer for nothing more than data storage. There is one *k*-space for each slice: 20 slices = 20 *k*-spaces; 30 slices = 30 *k*-spaces.

Echoes are placed in storage for the Fourier transform to work on when *k*-space has been filled. A *k*-space is thought to have three zones: The "center" and two "outer" zones. Each zone contributes to the image contrast and resolution.

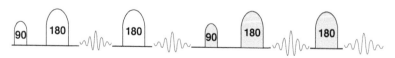

Figure 5.1 A multi echo (FSE/TSE) sequence.

Teaching Moment: The center zone contributes mostly to image contrast and SNR, and a little to resolution. The outer zones contribute more resolution or edge detail and only a little bit to image contrast (Figure 5.2).

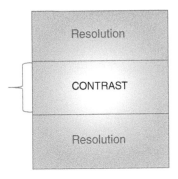

Figure 5.2 The center zone of *k*-space contributes close to 90% of an image's contrast. **You want the good TEs (effective TEs, ETEs) to be placed within the center lines.** They contribute the most to image contrast and SNR. The outer zones of *k*-space should be filled with the echoes that will contribute the least to image contrast. Outer zones contribute more to resolution or edge detail and less to image contrast.

A sequence is run with a desired contrast, the **effective TE (ETE)**, which comes from the TR/TE. In SE there is only one 180° so all the TEs are the same contrast. FSE has multiple echoes and therefore multiple contrasts are produced per TR that need to go into *k*-space. The ETEs tell the scanner which TEs go where. You want the **desired TEs** or ETEs placed in the **center** of *k*-space where they will contribute the most to the image **contrast**. Conversely, you want the least desirable TEs to be put into the outer zones. Putting certain echoes within certain zones of *k*-space happens by varying the amplitude of the phase encoding gradient (PEG)for each TE. **The ETE is always placed into the center zone of *k*-space.**

The decreased scan time from FSE is great, but we need think about what is happening. In FSE, the k-space for each slice is filled with different millisecond TEs, which is really a range of different contrasts.

Let us say, for example, you have a three-echo train: 10, 20, and 30 ms. One of those TEs will be selected as the desired contrast for the images, or the ETE.

You need to manage or concentrate those ETEs where they will do the most good for image contrast. The selected ETE tells the scanner to place those TEs in the center zone and others in the outer zones.

How to Place the ETEs

TEs are placed in the center or edges of k-space by varying the amplitude of the PEG that is applied to each echo in the ETL.

The **center zone** that contributes the most (90%) to image contrast and SNR and will get **a weaker amplitude PEG**. The **outer zones** will get **a stronger PEG applied**. These outer zones contribute mostly to the image's resolution or edge detail.

> **Teaching Moment:** Know that each zone contributes some contrast and resolution to the image, but the center gives more contrast and SNR than resolution, and the outer zones supply more resolution than contrast. This applies to all k-space and sequences.

Placing an echo in a different zone of k-space hinges upon the amplitude of the **PEG**. In FSE, the amplitude of the PEG changes for each echo. **High amplitudes** encode the echo to go into the **outer zones** for resolution, and **low amplitudes** put echoes in the **center** for contrast.

> **Teaching Moment:** The center zone gives you Contrast. Think: **C for C.**

The above high and low amplitude PEG playout is how image contrast is managed. (See Figure 5.6 for a visual depiction of the k-space filling just described.)

k-Space: Phase Encoding

When looking at a PSD, you will notice the PEG is often displayed as in Figure 5.3.

The lines or gradations in the diagram mean that the amplitude of the PEG is varied for each echo so the echo goes into a different zone of k-space. This varied PEG amplitude is in all pulse sequences. Figures 5.4 and 5.5 show varied amplitudes of the PEG.

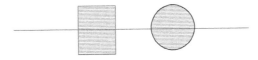

Figure 5.3 The phase encoding gradient (PEG).

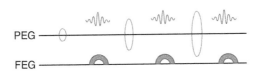

Figure 5.4 A weak amplitude PEG is applied to the first echo (ETE), putting it in the center zone (see also Figure 5.6).

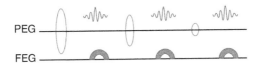

Figure 5.5 A low amplitude PEG is applied to the later echo (ETE) so it will be placed in the center zone (see also Figure 5.7).

Figure 5.6 *k*-Space is filled with ETE (10 ms) placed in the center by weak PEG. The other two echoes are placed in outer zones. See Figure 5.4. Resulting images will have the contrast of a 10 ms TE.

Figure 5.7 *k*-Space is filled as shown in Figure 5.5. The ETE (30 ms) is placed in the center by a weak amplitude PEG, with the other two echoes placed in outer zones by high amplitude PEGs. Images will have the contrast of a 30 ms TE.

With FSE, Watch the Speed Limit!

Saving time is great, but speed needs to be used for good. Remember that each 180° causes an echo which is farther away from the 90°. **The farther away from the 90°, the more T2 contrast. Each echo has to go into *k*-space.**

- If there are too many late echoes, i.e. T2 contrast, they can/will start to "outweigh" the center zone.

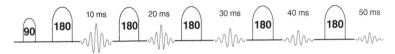

Figure 5.8 If the ETE is 10 ms, then the other four TEs will outweigh the first TE, making the resultant image look less T1 and have more T2 characteristics. An ETL of five is just too long for good T1 contrast. Also note that the amplitude of the echoes decreases as they get further away from the 90°.

- What is happening is that the T2 contrast starts to catch up to, and actually overcome, the T1 contrast.

On T1 weighted images, too large an ET will affect image contrast and IQ (Figure 5.8). Structures that are supposed to be dark on T1 (CSF) begin to brighten up (that is the T2 contrast coming through).

The longer the ETL, the more blur is seen in the image.

k-Space, ETL, and Image Contrast

Figure 5.9 shows how the center lines of *k*-space contribute to image contrast. If not enough center lines get filled with the ETE, IQ suffers.

Use TSE Speed for Good

Think about T1 weighting: Short TR and short TE.

Figure 5.8 shows an ETL of five. Echoes are acquired every 10 ms so you are acquiring echoes from 10 to 50 ms.

Teaching Moment: A 50 ms is not quite T2 but certainly not T1. Keep the ETL short for T1 contrast. All echoes must be placed into your *k*-space, and all echoes contribute something to image contrast and resolution.

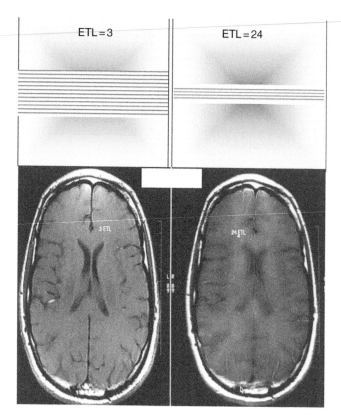

Figure 5.9 Taken at 3 T. Left. A 3 ETE of TE 10 ms. Decent T1 contrast, dark fluid, a little blur. Right. ETE of 10 ms, but with **ETL of 24** (ET from 10 to 240 ms) shows blur, and increased signal from CSF. TR also needed to be lengthened to accommodate the long ETL. The CSF is brightening in the sulci, as too many **T2 weighted** echoes got put into the *k*-space and crowded the center zone. On the right, there are fewer T1 contrast weighted lines and more T2 weighted lines. Also, it looks like the patient received gadolinium. Again, this is due to lots of T2 contrast getting into the *k*-space and overwhelming the T1 contrast. Also note the blurring from a long ETL.

General Rule. The maximum ETL for T1 contrast is three, four if you are desperate for shorter scan time. However, consider a previous statement, that all work uses a certain amount of TR. More echoes = longer TR (less T1), and more echoes = more T2 contrast. **But you want T1 contrast.** Having more than three echoes in a T1 is counterproductive. You are just making the images **less T1** by the longer TR or **more T2** with the long ETL.

Teaching Moment: Do not add T2 contrast to the k-space which is supposed to be T1 weighted (see Figure 5.9).

Some general numbers for ETLs:

- *T1:* **ETL of 2–4**. This keeps TR low and T2 out.
- *PD:* **ETL of 6–8**. Long TR keeps T1 out, and the shorter ETL keeps most T2 out.
- *T2:* **ETL of 18+**. This brings in T2, while long TR keeps T1 out.

Special Note on PD Weighting: Some radiologists want a long TR, 3500–4000 ms or higher, in order to eliminate as much T1 contrast as possible.

Filling *k*-Space

In Figure 5.10, note that the echoes in the center of k-space have higher amplitudes, which means a higher SNR than the outer zones. The center, again, contributes mostly to image contrast.

What else can we tell from this example of a SE k-space diagram? There are nine phase steps, so only nine TRs were needed to fill it. This will make more sense when you read about the scan time formula in Chapter 14.

Pros and Cons of FSE

- Time saver. Pro – **use it for good.**
- Multiple 180°s = decreased susceptibility artifacts: Pro.
- Increased SAR (ETL): Con.

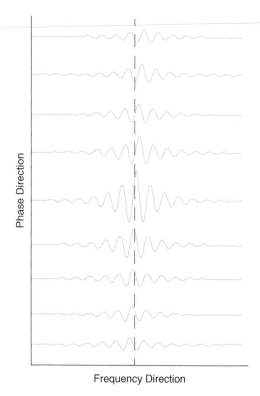

Figure 5.10 A very simplified depiction of a *k*-space. The scan matrix is 9 × 9: nine lines of phase and a frequency of nine. Each echo has the same frequency (9), but a different amount of phase. Each echo had a different amplitude PEG applied to it. The dashed line is used to show the different "phases" from echo to echo. The echoes cross the dashed line at different points when compared to each other.

- Decreased sensitivity to hemorrhage (ETL): Con.
- Brighter fat than expected (from ETL): Con.

Decreased sensitivity to hemorrhage/blood by-products and other magnetic susceptibilities comes from the ETL. This is both a Pro and a Con. The ETL makes the FSE one of the more artifact resistant sequences: Pro. Seeing blood is what GREs are for as they have no 180°s. FSEs have multiple 180°s so they clean up the effects of the hemoglobin: Con.

Teaching Moment: Be careful about using a multi-echo GRE sequence in the brain. The multi-echo portion of that sequence may decrease sensitivity to hemorrhage.

Increased SAR: Multiple 180°s equals lots of RF to the patient.
Brighter fat when compared to a conventional spin echo (CSE) sequence. This is due to something called "J-coupling," which is a quantum mechanics concept. A full explanation is outside of the realm of this book. However, J-coupling is how fat molecules interact with each other during excitation and relaxation. With all the refocusing pulses during an FSE, there will be some fat NMV in the X/Y plane at the TE.

Teaching Moment: NMVs pointing at the coil during the TE will be bright whether you want them to be or not. With the exception of cortical bone, air, or tendon/ligaments, nothing is ever totally dark or devoid of signal. If a tendon or ligament has some signal in it, it is pathology of some sort. There is always a small NMV from everything pointing toward the coil. This is why our images are "greyscale."

Another Way to View T2* and 180°s

Step back and re-think the T2/T2* curves from Chapter 3. This is a different way to understand T2* and the effects of a 180° on T2* in an FSE sequence.

- Question: What happens after the 90° or excitation pulse? If you said de-phasing or T2* you were correct.
- Question: What happens after the 180° causes an echo? If you said de-phasing or T2*, again you would be correct.

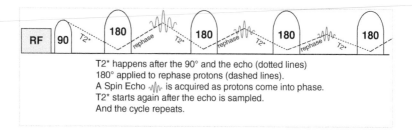

T2* happens after the 90° and the echo (dotted lines)
180° applied to rephase protons (dashed lines).
A Spin Echo ◦◦◦ is acquired as protons come into phase.
T2* starts again after the echo is sampled.
And the cycle repeats.

Figure 5.11 An FSE PSD with ETL of four. The 90° is followed by T2*, a 180° refocuses the T2* and a spin echo forms. T2* resumes, a 180° refocuses it, and another SE forms. This continues to the end of the echo train.

The de-phasing after the echo may be mentioned in text, but it is seldom if ever shown as a part of a line diagram. See Figure 5.11.

Teaching Moment: The amplitude of echoes decreases over time due to imperfections in the 180°'s RF and true T2 relaxation. Also remember that the further away from the 90° an echo is, the more T2 contrast is in the echo.

Where Do Relaxation and Decay Curves Come From?

The T1 relaxation and T2 decay curves come from a process of acquiring many data points of either T1 or T2 echoes over time, plotting them on a graph, and connecting the dots.

Figure 5.12A is an example of a T2* decay curve. Each dot in the line is a data point (echo) acquired over time in ms. The top left of the line shows TEs with high signal, and over time a signal intensity decays to zero (bottom right). If you connect each dot, a T2* relaxation curve is produced. It is a T2* curve as there are no 180°s involved.

What would the effect on this curve be, if a series 180° of RF pulses were applied and those TEs were to be plotted on a graph?

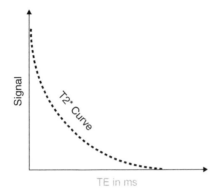

Figure 5.12A A T2* decay curve.

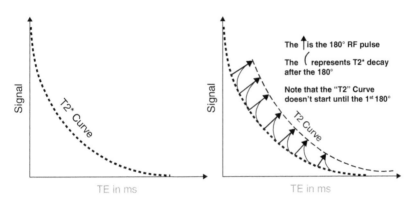

The ↑ is the 180° RF pulse

The (represents T2* decay after the 180°

Note that the "T2" Curve doesn't start until the 1st 180°

Figure 5.12A, B A. A T2* decay curve. B. A T2 decay curve.

A T2* Curve Compared to the T2 Curve

Here I am going to show you the effects of 180° RF pulses on a T2* decay curve. As soon as the 90° or excitation RF is turned off, **T2* starts.** De-phasing or T2* can and will be refocused by a 180°. If not refocused with 180°s, the T2* curve continues to decline until the signal drops to zero, as in Figure 5.12A. When the first 180° RF pulse is applied, de-phasing is reversed, SNR increases, and an SE results. That is your first data point.

De-phasing resumes, another 180°, another echo results and you have your second data point. The process continues to the end of the ETL (7). Now connect those data points and you get the **dashed line** as seen in Figure 5.12B: a T2 relaxation curve.

I show this comparison first to teach that there is such a thing as a T2* curve. They are not often mentioned, and seldom if ever compared to a T2 curve. If I showed you two decay curves, you would not be able to tell them apart.

Metal Artifact Reduction (MARS)

MARS is a technique on an FSE/SE to reduce the artifact caused by metal in or near the FOV. It is a generic technique or method that any system can do. Some vendors have specific software packages available designed to reduce the artifact from metal. I will not get specific here with vendors' names/terminology for their metal suppression software/techniques.

All you need to do is to edit the individual sequence parameters in your protocol to make it a "MARS." Think of saving it as a protocol for future use. It makes no sense working hard twice. There is no "MARS" button to push.

The Basic MARS Technique

Metal causes a very rapid de-phasing due to local field inhomogeneity. It also changes the precessional frequency of the protons in close proximity to the metal, making them un-imageable as it were. Metal actually speeds up the protons. Metal artifact is worse at 3 T, just like most other artifacts. There are several scan parameters you can change to decrease the effects of metal in the FOV:

- Increase the ETL (FSE only).
- Widen the bandwidth/Hz per pixel or narrow the water/fat separation.
- Use as small an FOV as possible.
- On T2s: use the shortest TE possible (e.g. 85 ms vs. 120 ms TE).

- On T1s: use the minimum TE (which you should be using anyway).
- Avoid GREs and fat-sat sequences: use STIR for fat suppression.

Driven Equilibrium: A "Forced T1"

What is driven equilibrium (DE)? It is sometimes called **Drive, Restore, or Fast Recovery** and it is **a way to get more T2 contrast** by forcing the protons to T1 so you can get T2 weighting with a shorter TR. It works because, at the end of the ETL, there will be some NMV leftover in the X/Y plane. Those leftovers are the long T1 relaxing tissues like edema, CSF, or urine.

There are two things you can do with the residual NMV:

1. Wait for it to T1 relax on its own which costs **time,** or
2. Use an RF pulse to make it T1 faster. How? Why?
    - If an RF pulse can push protons into the transverse plane, one can be used to push them back.
    - Remember, RFs are additive. A +90°RF followed by a +90°RF = 180°, but a +90°RF followed by a -90°RF = 0 (Figure 5.13). The extra 180° Drive pulse does not produce an echo. It just refocuses any residual NMV before it gets pushed back to 0° by the -90° RF pulse.

DE is used to get **increased signal from long T2 tissues (fluid).** It forces the long T1 tissues to T1 faster to get fluids ready for the next 90° RF pulse. Recall, fluids have long T1 and

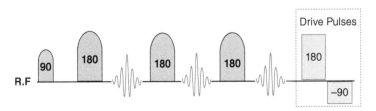

Figure 5.13 An FSE PSD with a driven equilibrium (DE) complex applied at the end of the ET. The DE complex is also known as Restore, Drive, or Fast Recovery.

T2 relaxation times. The DE pulses are placed at the end of the ET. The additional 180° RF puts everything back into phase, for the -90°RF to drive the NMV back into longitudinal. Remember, the initial excitation pulse is a + 90°. A **+90** followed by a **-90** = 0, essentially forcing the protons back to B_0 (see Figure 5.13).

Teaching Moment: Do not be confused by the idea of a forced T1. **This technique is absolutely not for use on T1 weighted images**. It is a **"forced T1"** in order to get more T2 contrast. If you try it on a T1 sequence, the CSF will get bright and you will get a phone call from a confused radiologist. See Figure 5.14 for an example of a T2 axial slice acquired with and without "Drive."

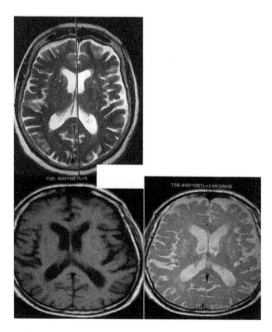

Figure 5.14 Top. **T2 axials** (split screen). Same patient, scan factors, and window levels on both sides. Left: Without Drive. Right: With Drive. Note the brighter CSF on the right. Bottom: **T1 axials**, left image without Drive and right image with Drive.

> **Driven Equilibrium: Summary:** A proton's nature is to return to its lowest energy state – **relaxation.**

Over time, a NMV will relax more and more. Eventually, the lowest energy state will be reached – **equilibrium.** Reaching equilibrium, however, takes time. The mechanism to speed up the process of reaching equilibrium is generically called **driven equilibrium.**

Why Use DE?

- Can save you time: Pro.
- May help get you more slices: Pro.
- Helps to increase T2 contrast: Pro.
- Increased SAR: Con.
- Cannot be used on all weightings: Semi-Con.

You absolutely cannot use DE on T1s but it can be used on PD, Short Time Inversion Recovery (STIR), and T2s. All three give you bright fluid. DE makes the fluid brighter.

> **Vendor-specific Names:**
>
> - FR: Fast Recovery: GE.
> - Restore: Siemens.
> - Drive: Philips.
> - DE-FSE: Hitachi.

3D FSE: CUBE/SPACE/VISTA

These are relatively new sequences (Figure 5.15). Most vendors have them and a big plus for using them is that they are 3D, meaning that they can be MIP'd and Multi-Planar Reformatted (MPR'd). Some vendors also offer a T1 weighted 3D FSE. 3Ds

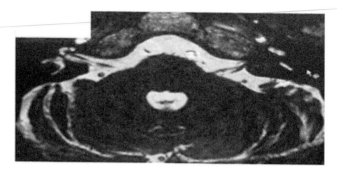

Figure 5.15 Image obtained from 3D axial FSE, commonly known as "CUBE" or "SPACE," which is frequently used in cranial nerve studies where high-resolution images are key.

will give you higher resolution over a 2D from very thin slices. These 3D sequences have long ETLs (>100 for T2s). You would expect the SNR on the late echoes to be very low but that is not the case. **The 180° RF pulses in 3D TSE are modified or modulated, which does a few good things:**

- There is less SAR than you would expect with a large ETL.
- Blurring is lessened with these long ETLs.
- SNR is higher in the late echoes compared to 2D sequences without the modified RF pulses. The modified 180°s slow down T2 decay so SNR is increased on late echoes.

Single Shot FSE/HASTE

Another variation of an FSE is called HASTE (Half Fourier Acquired Single Shot Turbo Spin Echo). Single shot FSE (SSFSE) and single shot TSE (SSTSE) are Echo Planar Imaging (EPI)-FSE techniques.

The term "single shot" means that all lines of k-space are filled following a single 90° excitation RF. This also means that the ETL is 128–256, maybe even more. You would surmise that an ETL of 128 would have significant blurring and very low signal by the end of that ETL. To combat this, k-space is filled in in reverse. This reversal puts the early echoes with the most SNR and least blur on the edges of k-space, and late echoes (with the most blur) in the center for their contrast. Recall that the outer lines of k-space contribute mostly to image resolution.

There is another way to speed things up. An SSFSE can use something called "partial Fourier." This is a modification of the **Fourier transformation** method. It is known that raw data in k-space is symmetric, or has symmetry. We can take advantage of that symmetry to decrease scan times. Symmetry of k-space (Hermitian symmetry) is a basic property of the **Fourier transform**. Partial or half-Fourier is also known as "phase conjugate synthesis." Half-Fourier works by acquiring only a little over half (60%) of k-space and sort of "copy-pasting" or synthesizing the rest. This means that once the k-space is a little over half full, a pattern can be determined and the rest of the data is synthesized, making the entire image possible at very short scan times.

Symmetry of k-Space: Phase Conjugate Synthesis

In mathematics, phase conjugate synthesis of a number means that a number with a real (scanned) part has an imaginary (synthesized or interpolated) part of equal and opposite value. The phase conjugate of $5 + 7x$ is $5 - 7x$. Here are some examples:

1. Simply put, k-space is a mirror image of itself with equal and equal and opposite values on the opposing side.
2. Figure 5.16 displays that the "K" (our k-space) on the right is a mirror opposite of the left.
3. Figure 5.17 shows a value top left has equal and opposite value top right. Bottom left is equal and opposite to bottom right.

While the above may be oversimplified, Figure 5.18 should hopefully bring the idea of symmetry home. Figure 5.18 shows that just over 50% of k-space is filled, which is enough to discern

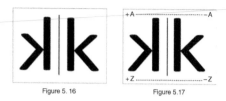

Figure 5. 16   Figure 5.17

Figure 5.16 and 5.17 *k*-Space is symmetrical and is a mirror image of itself, from left to right and even top to bottom.

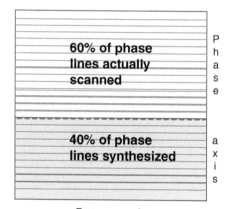

Frequency axis

Figure 5.18 Half-Fourier *k*-space filling. A little more than half of the lines in the phase direction are scanned (top lines). Bottom grey areas are those lines that are not scanned but synthesized. Scan time decreases by ≈ 40%, but SNR drops about 20–30%. Resolution will also decrease as some outer lines are not filled with real data. **There is just no substitute for real data.**

the symmetric pattern in *k*-space. Once that is established, the rest of *k*-space can be synthesized allowing Fourier transform to calculate the images.

Partial or half-Fourier examples are shown in Figure 5.19.

HASTE/SS-FSE/SS-TSE

HASTE or "single shots" are a combination of EPI and FSE. The ET acquired is not a typical "RF" ET, but an ET from a series of frequency gradient reversals.

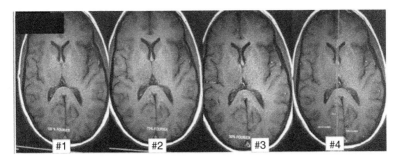

Figure 5.19 The effect on resolution and SNR with increasing half or partial Fourier factors. Sampling less lines of k-space to save time is great but it has its consequences. With fewer lines of real data going into k-space, IQ, in SNR and resolution, suffers. Again, there is just no substitute for real data. #1 is 100% k-space filled, #2 is 75%, and #3 is 50%. #4 is a split screen with 100% on the left and 50% on the right. Note loss of SNR and resolution as partial Fourier percentages are increased.

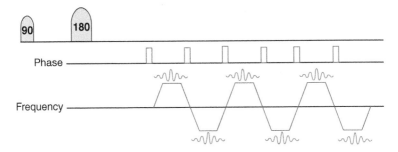

Figure 5.20 SSPSD. A single 90–180° RF pulse excites a slice. PEG is "blipped" on for each echo. Each additional phase application adds to the previous one, putting echoes in a different line of k-space. Note a series of FEG reversals.

In SS imaging there is one 90°/180° RF complex putting the NMV into the X/Y plane for a particular slice. Phase encoding is done with a series of "blipped" gradient applications, one for each frequency reversal. A long series of FEG reversals follows (the EPI part of it) (Figure 5.20). Each reversal causes an echo, and each echo fills a line of k-space (Figures 5.21 and 5.22). In order to keep the number of acquired phase lines low (avoiding blur), a partial Fourier technique is used which, as previously

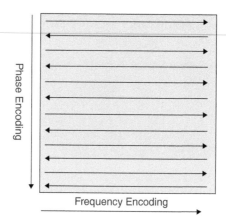

Figure 5.21 Trajectory *k*-space filling in SSFSE. Note lines of *k*-space filling from left/right, then right/left, then left/right, right/left. This "trajectory" filling is due to FEG reversals.

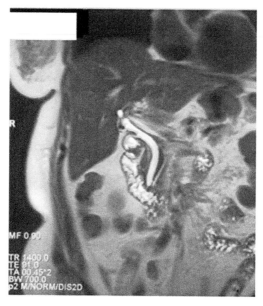

Figure 5.22 Coronal T2 weighted SSFSE.

explained, uses the symmetry in *k*-space to fill in the "un-filled" lines. Once done with slice 1, the scanner moves on to slice 2, and when it is done with 2, moves on to number 3 – a sequential pattern. These are T2 weighted images owing to their long ETs.

Single shots, by virtue of the way *k*-space is filled, do not have a TR per se. The definition of TR is the time from one 90° to the next 90° that excites the same slice, but in SS we do not go back to any slice. Each slice is excited once and then that slice is done. A TR of 10,000 ms may be displayed but that is not totally accurate. SSs should not be confused with FSE/TSEs. Conventional FSEs are by nature "multi-shots," meaning that there are many "TRs" per slice with each TR filling multiple lines of *k*-space whereas SSs fill all lines of phase for a slice in a single TR.

Thoughts on Acquiring HASTE

▩ Ideally these should be acquired in **sequential order**: 1, 2, 3, 4 for the first breath-hold, then 5, 6, 7, 8 for the second breath-hold. Why?

▩ Have you ever noticed that on coronals, the liver is up, then down, then up again? That is because slices are not being acquired sequentially. Try it, you will like it.

▩ What sequential acquisition order means is that all the lines of *k*-space are filled for slice 1, then for slice 2, then for slice 3, then for slice 4. See a pattern?

▩ Sequential acquisitions are important on axial breath holds because if the patient's breathing varies (is inconsistent) in theory you could miss every other slice (half the liver). The radiologists will not be happy.

▩ Sequential is more for aesthetics on coronals, but on axials it is about **not missing anatomy.** Why axials?

▩ On axials, you are imaging in the same direction as the anatomy is moving with respiration. Anatomy is moving, and the slices are moving as well with more than one acquisition. Two moving objects are going to miss each other unless you are on a highway during rush hour.

▩ Try an SSFSE respiratory triggered sequence. Overall scan time is a bit longer but they are very nice.

▩ SSFSEs are mostly used for heavy T2 weighting like MRCPs, Scouts/Localizers, and non-breath-hold abdominal sequences.

▩ SSFSE has a high temporal resolution (it scans very fast).

Notes

6

Tissue Suppression

Chapter at a Glance

MRI Physics: Tech to Tech Explanations, First Edition. Stephen J. Powers.
© 2021 John Wiley & Sons Ltd. Published 2021 by John Wiley & Sons Ltd.

IR Prepped Sequences
  IR Prepped Pulses
How is an RF Pulse Selective or Non-Selective?
Water Excitation Sequences

So far, I have talked about getting signal from tissues and how contrast is vital. Now I shall start to discuss how to **not** to get signal from select tissues and how this can and will alter the image contrast. In MR we can selectively choose to saturate a tissue so that it gives little to no signal, or we can suppress a tissue's signal. The methods of suppression vs. saturation are different but give the same result – less signal from our target tissue. The vast majority of the time, fat will be the target tissue.

There is a difference between **suppression** and **saturation**. **Saturation** means targeting a particular tissue with **RF** pulse to diminish its signal. That tissue is exposed to RF pulses tuned to the tissue's particular precessional frequency (PF) in order to saturate (overexpose if you like) the tissue prior to slice excitation. Recall earlier that I said a tissue needs to be able to T1 relax (stand up) after RF excitation. The saturation technique is a series of 90° RF pulses, followed very quickly by the 90–180°, so 90°, 90°, 90°, then 90–180°. The three quick 90°s set up something called the "steady state" in the target tissue.

Steady state basically means that a tissue has not had time to T1 relax, nor is it pushed back into the X/Y plane any further.

Targeting a specific tissue for saturation is sometimes referred to as **"chemical saturation."** Why the word "chemical"? While fat and water both contain lots of hydrogen, they have different molecular structures, so are really different chemicals. Both fat and water have their own precessional frequency, which we can and will take advantage of.

Let us assume we are saturating fat on an FSE. Fat gets three quick 90° RF pulses, resulting in its NMV being in a steady state with a very small transverse NMV. At TE, fat with a very small transverse NMV gives very little signal. There are two drawbacks or issues with fat saturation (fat-sat): The patient's SAR is increased (a concern at 3 T), and sometimes the scanner has difficulty tuning for fat-sat, especially when imaging away from isocenter.

Tissue suppression lowers a tissue's signal by another means, an Inversion Pulse (a 180° RF that pushes the Longitudinal NMV from 0° past 90° and down to 180°). The 180° inversion recovery (IR) pulse is not tuned to a tissue-specific frequency like a fat-sat pulse is. Basically, what happens is, all tissues with similar T1 relaxation times will be suppressed.

Tissue Saturation versus Suppression

In the IR scenario, you are **suppressing** signal from a tissue by virtue of its T1 relaxation rate. IR Sequences actually suppress all tissues with similar T1 relaxations.

IR sequences have been a staple in MRI for years. As soon as you hear "IR," think an RF pulse with a delay time after it called the "TI" or Time of Inversion. It is stated in ms. There are two forms of IRs: **STIR** and **FLAIR**. Both of these sequences are basically the same with a couple of minor differences.

- *STIR: Short Time (or TAU) Inversion Recovery.*
- *FLAIR: Fluid Attenuated Inversion Recovery.* There are two kinds of FLAIRs:
  - T1 FLAIR: Long TR, short TE, and intermediate TI.
  - T2 FLAIR: Very long TR, long TE, and long TI.

In an IR, the TI is key for which tissue gets suppressed.

Teaching Moment: Short TIs suppress short (fast) T1 relaxing tissue: **fat, gadolinium, and protein**. The opposite is true. Long TIs suppress long (slow) T1 relaxing tissue: **CSF**.

IR sequences have a simple PSD: It is basically an SE that starts with a 180° inversion pulse, then the 90/180° RFs typical for an SE. The inversion pulse is an RF pulse that excites the entire slice. **The TI allows tissues to T1 to the "null" point**.

Remember, fat is fast to T1, fluid is slow to T1, is key.

Inversion Recovery – Part One: STIR

Let us begin with STIR. Know that in Inversion Recovery sequences, it is all about the TI.

A STIR PSD starts with a 180° pulse to invert the NMV (Figure 6.1). After the 180°, time is given for tissue to T1 relax. During the TI, fat, with a short T1, relaxes faster than fluids do, so most of the fat NMV is at the **"null point"** at the end of the TI. What is the "null point"? Think of it as the X/Y or transverse plane. **What "null" means is that at the end of the TI, whatever tissue is in the X/Y plane – whether it is fat, gadolinium, protein, or CSF – will be nulled (suppressed).**

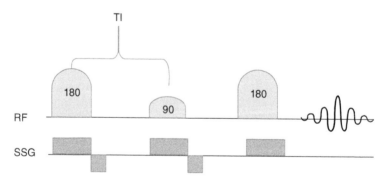

Figure 6.1 A basic IR PSD. What is happening during the TI is T1 relaxation. Fat, gadolinium, and protein are fast and will be suppressed by a short TI. CSF is slow and will be suppressed by a long TI.

At the end of the TI, a 90° RF is applied to the slice. **Remember, RFs are additive**. So, if fat is at the null point (90°) and another 90° comes that is 90° + 90° = 180° so fat's NMV gets knocked back down to the longitudinal (away from the coil) and will not give signal at TE. Water's NMV (slow to T1) is mostly still at 180°. The 90° comes in and forces water to 270° (pointing at the coil). The next 180° flips water's NMV over, still pointing at the coil, so water gives signal at TE. This is why fluid/edema is bright on a STIR.

Inversion Recovery: STIR with Vectors

$$180°\text{TI} \rightarrow 90° \rightarrow 180° \rightarrow \text{TE}$$

The STIR sequence is shown in Figures 6.2 to 6.7.

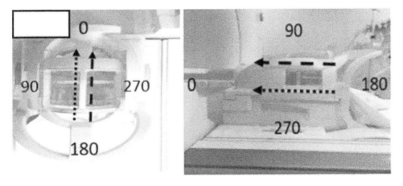

Figure 6.2 The NMVs shown are **pre** 180° inversion pulse. The dashed arrow represents the fat NMV, the dotted arrow the NMV of fluid. NMV positions change as result of the RF pulses.

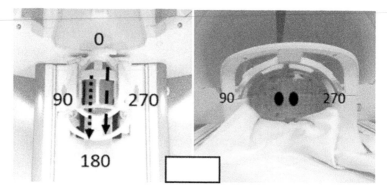

Figure 6.3 NMVs **post** 180° RF. On the right, looking up the bore, NMV is pointing at you as represented by the dots.

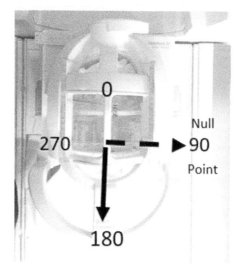

Figure 6.4 During the TI, fat T1 relaxes to the null point with water pretty much still inverted at 180. Remember tissue at the **null point** when the TI runs out will ultimately be suppressed or "nulled."

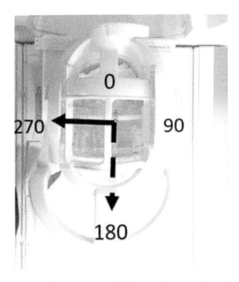

Figure 6.5 After the of the TI, a 90° is applied to the slice, driving fat (dashed line) back to 180°, and water (solid line), which was at 180°, is driven to 270°. Remember, RF pulse can add to the NMV. So, an NMV at +90° that receives another +90° is driven to 180°, 180 + 90 = 270.

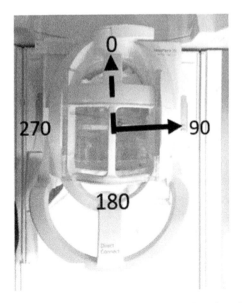

Figure 6.6 The 180° is the final RF pulse applied to the slice, driving fat (dashed line) to 0°. Water (solid line), which was at 270°, is driven to 90° (X/Y). Water's NMV is pointing at the coils at TE.

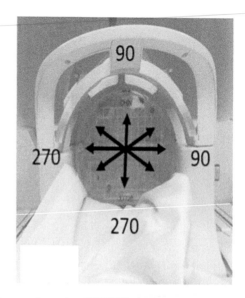

Figure 6.7 Remember, the 90°/270° position is the transverse plane, and the NMV is a rotating vector spinning like an airplane propeller. The resulting NMV positions are as follows. Fat (a fast T1 tissue) is at 0°, **generating no signal** by not pointing at the coil. Water/fluids are in the X/Y plane and pointing at the coil at the TE generating signal. Here you are looking up the bore at the coil, which shows the coil positioned around the phantom in the X/Y or transverse plane. Vectors in this plane are rotating and pointing at the coil, generating signal.

Teaching Moment: An Image Quality Question: STIR can be a long sequence. There is extra TR built in. **You need to keep it.** The extra TR is in there for a reason. The extra TR gives long T1 tissue (fluids) time to T1 relax. Resist the urge to drop the TR to save time. That can saturate the very tissues you want to see: CSF/edema (Figure 6.8). These are long T1 tissues that need the long TR in order to T1 and be seen.

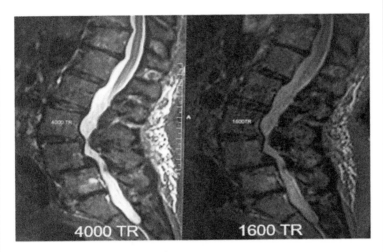

Figure 6.8 Two STIR images. The one on the right was scanned at 1600 ms TR, the one on the left was scanned at 4000 ms TR. Same slice and same patient. Fat is still suppressed as you would expect from the TI. That is not the problem. The issue is the lack of signal from CSF and marrow edema. The right image is just not a good STIR. CSF is saturated as the TR was too short and it did not have enough time to T1 relax. The left image is the better of the two.

Inversion Recovery Part Two: T2 FLAIR

The T2 FLAIR sequence has the same basic PSD as a STIR (see Figure 6.1) but with two differences: The TI and the TE. The FLAIR sequence's long TI is used to suppress CSF in the brain. A long TE makes it T2 weighted.

The timing of the RF pulses causes the NMV of CSF to be suppressed just like fat in a STIR. A long TI suppresses long T1 relaxing tissue. I shall quickly go through the NMV positions.

- The 180° inverts both fat and CSF.
- During the TI, CSF relaxes to the null point (90°) and fat, because it is fast, gets all the way to 0°.

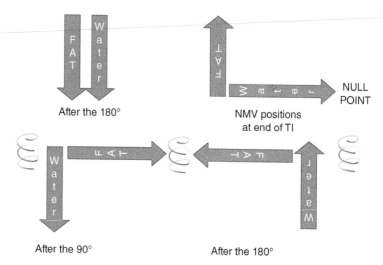

Figure 6.9 A pictogram of water and fat NMV positions from the RF pulses during a T2 FLAIR. These are the same as those in a STIR. The tissues are just opposite. The final 180° RF puts the NMV of short T1 tissue to the X/Y plane and pointing at the coil to give signal. The NMV of CSF is in the longitudinal, not pointing at the coil, so unable to give signal. T2 FLAIRs are used almost exclusively in the brain to suppress CSF. Edema from tumors, infections, and multiple sclerosis has different T1 times so will be in the X/Y plane at TE. Edema actually has a shorter T1 time than CSF and acts more like fat (both bright) due to the chemical makeup.

- The 90° pushes CSF to 180° (remember, 90 + 90 = 180) and fat and other fast T1 tissues go to 90°.
- Lastly, the 180° pushes the CSF vector to 0°, and the fat to 270°, the X/Y or transverse plane.
- So, fat and other short T1 tissues will be pointing at the coil, generating signal. Figure 6.9 demonstrates the NMV's direction as a result of the different RF pulses.
- Stop and look at a T2 next to a T2 FLAIR. A T2 FLAIR is just a T2 with dark fluid. Both have the same grey/white matter characteristics.

I have already said this, but it bears repeating: **Long** TIs will suppress **long** T1 tissue, **short** TIs will suppress **short** T1 tissue. FLAIR and STIR are compared in Figures 6.10 and 6.11.

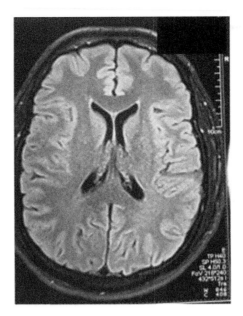

Figure 6.10 T2 FLAIR. CSF is dark and shows similar T2 contrast differences between Grey Matter and White Matter similar to those seen in a conventional T2 weighted FSE. T2 FLAIR sequence: Long TR to decrease T1, long TE to increase T2, and a long TI to suppress CSF.

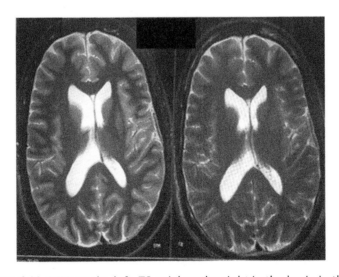

Figure 6.11 STIR on the left, T2 axial on the right in the brain in the same patient. Both demonstrate dark fat and bright CSF. Uses of STIR in the brain are usually for suppressing fat in the orbits and in pediatric exams. Children are not well myelinated so getting good GM/WM contrast is difficult. STIR gives you that GM/WM differentiation as WM, with a short T1 from its high lipid content, is suppressed. However, STIR is much more motion sensitive.

> **Teaching Moment:** Large FOVs benefit from STIR over fat-sat as big FOVs have more inhomogeneities causing inconsistent fat-sat in the FOV.

IR Sequences: T1 and T2 FLAIR

All IR sequences use the same 180°, 90°, 180° scheme of RF pulses. The differences are in the TI and TE: a shorter TI and a short TE on a T1 FLAIR. Already you may have thought a short TE equals less T2. The TR is much longer than expected in FSE to accommodate the TI. So, why the TR, TE, TI differences between T2/T1 FLAIR?

First, TE differences are for T1 vs. T2 contrast. The TRs and TIs need to have a ratio between them. In T2 FLAIR, the TR needs to be four times the TI, and for T1, the TR should be three times the TI. Most scanners now have "Auto TI" turned on so if the TR is changed, the TI changes automatically. No math is needed on your part. The ratio between the TR and TI is not exact. We are not going to Pluto on the numbers, but they should be pretty close.

T1 FLAIRs can be run post gadolinium. It is common for sites to do this, especially at 3 T, where getting good T1 contrast can be a challenge.

Tissue suppression in IRs is not "tissue specific," meaning that an IR pulse inverts all tissue in the slice whereas in fat-sat only fat gets excited with an RF pulse tuned to the PF of fat. In IR all tissues with similar T1 relaxation times get suppressed:

- *STIR:* Fat, gadolinium, protein.
- *FLAIR:* Long TI suppresses long T1 tissue: CSF and urine (Figure 6.12).

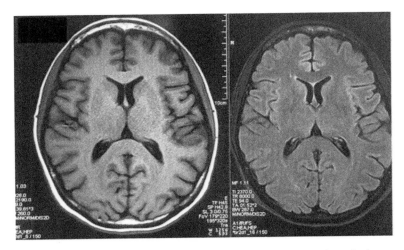

Figure 6.12 Same slice, same patient. Left. The T1 FLAIR has dark CSF and good GM/WM differentiation just like in T1 FSE. Right. The T2 FLAIR shows CSF dark and the same T2 contrast differences between GM and WH as seen in T2 FSE. Also notice that on the T2 FLAIR, the darker WM allows abnormal WM (as in MS) to show as bright pericallosal spots/dots. T2 FLAIRs are often fat-sat.

FLAIR Factors (scan factors not empirical):

- *T2 FLAIR:* TR 8500–9500, TI 2200–2500, TE 120+ ms.
- *T1 FLAIR:* TR 2500–3000, TI 800–900, TE 10–20 ms.

IR Weightings: STIR, T1 and T2 FLAIR

What is the weighting of STIRs vs. FLAIRs? Let's do **STIR** first.

- STIR has bright fluid and dark fat, which is opposite to a T1 with bright fat and dark fluid. Not sounding T1, is it?
- STIR has bright fluid and dark fat, T2 has bright fluid with bright-ish fat. STIR is not exactly T2 contrast either.

- STIR and T2 fat-sat look similar with dark fat and bright fluid. There are very similar contrasts from both. The fat suppression comes from a different mechanism. Sounds T2 weighted.
- *Answer:* STIR is T1 weighted. Tissue suppression is based on the **T1 relaxation time** of fat. The TI used is based on the T1 of fat. All tissue with similar T1 relaxation times to fat will suppress. Gadolinium and proteins fit the description.

Signal suppression with STIR, being based on T1 relaxation times, is not tissue specific like fat-sat. This means that multiple tissues can be suppressed by a single TI: Fat, gadolinium, and proteins. STIR is often used for bone marrow pathology whereas T2 fat-sat is frequently used in soft tissue injury/pathology. That is not a rule, but is common to many protocols. There is also a radiologist preference. Some like STIR over a T2 fat-sat. STIR is more motion sensitive, but less sensitive to offset FOVs and field inhomogeneities like metal. STIR is a go-to sequence if there is metal in the FOV. It has similar contrast to T2 fat-sat.

What about T1 and T2 FLAIRs? What is their weighting? **T1 FLAIR** is T1 weighted from relatively short TR and TE to decrease T2 contrast. The TI suppresses CSF. Look at Figure 6.12. It has good GM/WM contrast like a T1 SE, and dark CSF as it was targeted to be dark by the TI. **T2 FLAIR** is T2 from long TR/TEs to increase T2. The long TI suppresses CSF. There is similar GM/WM contrast as in a T2 (dark WM, bright-ish GM). It has T2 contrasts, just with dark fluid.

Where do those "TIs" come from?: Without all kinds of graphs and line diagrams, the TIs you commonly use are derived from some pretty simple math. If you know the T1 time of a tissue, any tissue, multiply that by 0.69 and the answer is the TI that will suppress it. The T1 of fat at 1.5 T is ≈220 ms ($220 \times 0.69 = 151$) and at 3 T it is ≈280 ms ($280 \times 0.69 = 193$). The same is true for CSF/FLAIR. The T1 time of CSF is multiplied by 0.69 and that is the TI for CSF.

Teaching Moment: A STIR trick. If fat is too dark, drop the TI by, say, 20–30 ms; if not dark enough, increase by 20–30 ms. Think of the TI as fat suppression control (Figure 6.13).

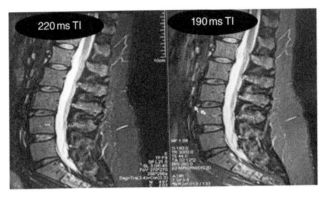

Figure 6.13 Left. Increased TI = darker, 220 ms. Right. Decreased TI = lighter, 190 ms. Note darker subcutaneous fat and bone marrow on left image.

Inversion Recovery – Part Two

My previous explanation on IR, while easier to understand visually, does not give the real story. While the 180° inverts the NMV (spins it down), its path back to B_0 does not actually spin back up to cross the X/Y or 90° plane. It goes back up from 180° to 0° like an elevator. Straight up. It has no transverse component at 180° so takes the path of least resistance. Most depictions of T1 curves show the starting off point as the 90° or transverse plane. They are true for everything except an IR sequence. An IR's T1 curve starting point is at the 180°. A T1 curve is a T1 curve but in IR it just starts off from a different point, 180°. In Figure 6.14, the curve represents the amount of T1 that has gone back up to 0° during the TI. As it passes through the "null point" (think of it as the X/Y plane), a 90° RF is applied and that tissue will be "nulled." **Tissues relaxing faster (those that got above**

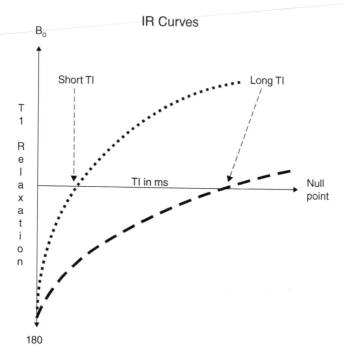

Figure 6.14 Relaxation starts off at 180° and progresses towards the null point. The dotted line is fat. It relaxes fast, so a short TI hits it at the null point: **dark fat, bright fluid.** The dashed line is fluid. It is slow to T1 so a long TI catches it at its null point: **dark fluid, bright fat.**

the null point) or relaxing slower (below the null point) when the 90° is applied will not be suppressed.

The Rupture View

When a patient has silicone breast implants, they can rupture either naturally or from trauma. Postoperatively, a capsule of scar tissue forms around the implant, and if the implant ruptures, the plastic membrane containing the silicone collapses onto itself and the silicone is contained solely by the scar tissue. The collapsed membrane can look like spaghetti on the images – the "linguini" sign.

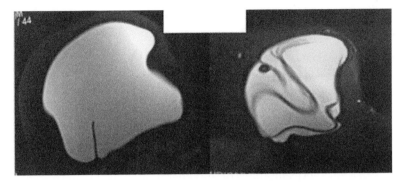

Figure 6.15 Two different implants. The one on the left is intact but with a fold, which is not uncommon. On the right is a ruptured implant showing the "linguini" sign. 3000 TR, 40 TE TI = 150.

The "rupture view" is an IR (STIR) used to suppress two different tissues at once: Fat and water. This sequence has a short TI and a water saturation pulse. A STIR sequence can have a **water saturation** pulse and TI for **fat suppression**. This combination of TI and pre-excitation leaves only silicone able to give signal at TE. Bright silicone is desired as the membrane that has collapsed will be dark. Figure 6.15 demonstrates a ruptured implant. Silicone is bright, breast tissue (fat) and implant liner are dark. You only want signal from silicone. Of additional concern in a traumatic implant rupture is silicone migration outside of the capsule of scar tissue.

Tissue Saturation: Chemical Shift

Everything – fat, water, muscle, etc. – each has its own PF, and 99% of the time we are saturating fat. We can take advantage of the PF differences, especially at high field strengths. The difference in PF between tissues is often referred to as "chemical shift." Let's saturate fat. At the higher fields PF differences between fat and water increases. They are 220 Hz at 1.5 T to 440 Hz at 3 T. At lower fields, say below 1 T, the differences are much less and getting chemical saturation is difficult. Figure 6.16 shows that the space between peaks, or chemical shift, is larger

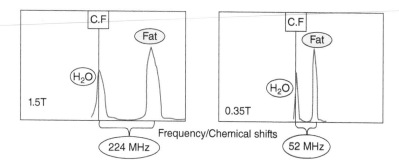

Figure 6.16 Representations of the separation of the fat and water peaks (chemical shift) at two different field strengths: 1.5 T and 0.35 T. C.F. = Center frequency.

at 1.5 T than it is at 0.35 T. Because of this, a fat-sat pulse at 0.35 T can and will also pre-excite some water and overall SNR suffers. A fat-sat at 3 T is easy due to the large chemical shift.

Fat-sat: Fat-sat causes higher SAR from the extra RF pulses and more work for the scanner. You may need a longer TR again to accommodate the extra RF pulses. Extra work = extra TR. **Be careful for too long of a TR in T1 land.**

So, you may have memorized the numbers for the differences in PF as: 3.5 ppm, 224 Hz at 1.5 T and 444 Hz at 3 T (rounded to give or take a few Hz). Those numbers are the "stock" answers if and when asked.

- The difference between fat and water is **3.5 ppm**, no matter what field strength. It is a constant.
- What does the 3.5 ppm mean? It means that for every 1 million (1,000,000.0) rotations that water does, fat does 3.5 less or 999,996.5 rotations (1,000,000 - 3.5).
- If water does 2,000,000 rotations, fat does 1,999,993.0. You can see that as water speeds up, so too does fat, just not as much. Fat lags behind.

▣ What about the **220** and **440**? Those numbers come from a simple equation: The Larmor frequency × 3.5 = the PF difference. They are directly proportional to field strength. So:

Water	Fat
■ 63.85 MHz × 3.5	= 223 Hz less
■ 127.71 MHz × 3.5	= 445 Hz less
■ 29.79 MHz × 3.5	= 104.2 Hz less (at 0.7 T).

Why is fat a slower PF? Simple. Fat is a big molecule and water is small. Fat is a long string of hydrocarbons. An aircraft carrier (fat) just cannot go as fast as a cigar racing boat (water).

Chemical Saturation at Low Fields

The PF difference at higher fields is bigger, while at lower fields it is less. As the PF difference gets larger, it is easier to take advantage of the chemical shift and get good fat-sat. This is the main reason why fat-sat at low fields is difficult to almost impossible: The chemical shift is too small to take advantage of. At low fields, **STIR** and **Dixon** sequences give a more reliable form of fat-sat.

▣ **STIR** does not care about PF differences. STIR cares about the T1 of the tissue to be suppressed. As long as you have the correct TI, it suppresses. The T1 time of a tissue × 0.69 = the TI to suppress it.

▣ **Dixon** is a GRE sequence that acquires an in and out of phase TE then does a series of calculations to give you not only in and out of phase echoes, but a "water only" data set, which means you only get signal from water-containing structures so for all intents and purposes it is a fat-sat. The "fat only" images mean you are only seeing signal from fat-containing structures. It looks like breast images when you have missed the water peak and do not get good fat suppression. FYI, a tissue's PF has nothing to do with its T1 relaxation time. Fat has a lower PF compared to water, but a short T1 relaxation. Water has a higher PF, but long T1. There is more information on the Dixon sequence later in this chapter.

Tissue Saturation: SPAIR and SPIR

These two signal suppression methods use a combination of IR and fat-sat: SPAIR (spectral attenuation IR) and SPIR (spectral pre-saturation IR). You may have guessed that the "IR" means an inversion recovery type sequence. SPAIR and SPIR are very similar to STIR sequences. The difference is the IR pulse; while both start off with an IR (180°) pulse, **the 180° is specifically tuned to the PF of fat**. The 180°s in STIR/FLAIR are wide B/W RFs, meaning they are not "tissue specific," whereas in SPAIR and SPIR they are tissue specific.

- In **SPAIR**, the 180° is an "adiabatic" pulse. Adiabatic is a type of RF pulse that is better in non-uniform RF fields. It more precisely inverts fat's NMV and generates less heat. The 180° is applied multiple times during the TR to suppress any T1 that fat may have occurred. There is no user-selectable TI in SPAIR.
- **SPIR** combines an IR pulse of 100–180° followed by a spoiler gradient to null fat. SPIR has an adjustable TI.

Unlike STIR/FLAIR (which is its own sequence), SPAIR/SPIR are preparatory RF pulses that can be added to a sequence (like fat-sat, they can be turned on/off) and are alternatives to fat-sat where large FOV, large offsets, or other causes of field inhomogeneities affect IQ. Both SPAIR and SPIR target fat for suppression; STIR is a non-selective tissue suppressor.

Tissue Saturations: STIR, T1 and T2 SPAIR: The short TI in STIR suppresses short T1 tissue: fat, gadolinium, and protein. SPAIR and SPIR have higher SNR and can be used post gadolinium, unlike STIR (Figure 6.17).

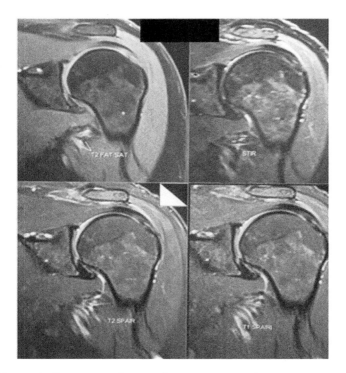

Figure 6.17 A series of same slice, same patient images at 1.5 T where all geometric factors were maintained. Top left. A T2 fat-sat has good signal uniformity and resolution. Top right. STIR also has equal image contrasts and signal uniformity. STIR has the lowest resolution of the four. Bottom left. A T2 with the option of SPAIR enabled. Note slightly better resolution (less blur) and very good signal uniformity. Bottom right. T1, SPAIR turned on. T1 SPAIR can be done post IV contrast.

Review: Fat-sat and SPAIR/SPIR target fat for saturation. Fat-sat uses a 90° RF pulse tuned to fat's PF while SPAIR and SPIR use 180°s tuned to fat. STIR/FLAIR uses a wide-bandwidth 180° inversion pulse, meaning it is not tissue specific. Depending on the TI, all tissues with a short or long T1 relaxation will be suppressed. **Fat-sat, SPAIR, and SPIR's** contrasts come from **PF differences**, whereas **STIR/FLAIR** contrasts are **T1 relaxation based.**

The Dixon Technique

The Dixon technique has been around for years. It was developed/described in 1984 by W. Thomas Dixon while scanning on a 0.35 T. The Dixon technique is neither a saturation nor a suppression technique. It is used mostly for fat suppression on low fields for the following reason: at low fields, the "chemical shift" between fat and water is rather small, meaning the peaks are much closer together than at higher fields. With small chemical shift, some of the fat-sat pulse also suppresses water signal so SNR drops. The Dixon technique acquires in and out of phase echoes (IP and OOP TEs). It then uses them to mathematically eliminate signal from either fat or water.

The Dixon technique needs rather precise IP and OOP TEs. If they are off, the math starts to fail and IQ will suffer. Suffice it to say, the actual equations will make your head spin so they are not stated here; they are, however, in Chapter 14: "MRI Math."

The Dixon technique is **relatively** insensitive to inhomogeneities of B_0 and B_1 and while it is not a "metal artifact suppression option" it is a bit more forgiving than the conventional fat-sat technique. Again, in the presence of metal, and when bright fluid/dark fat is needed, STIR is the sequence of choice due to its relative insensitivity to metal.

The Dixon technique acquires IP and OOP TEs to do a series of math problems which will produce four sets of images: in phase, out of phase, **water only** and **fat only**. There are several vendor-specific names for the Dixon technique (GE: Ideal; Siemens: Dixon; Hitachi: Fat-Sep). Some vendors offer the choice to get all four sets or just the water or fat only images. Figure 6.18 shows all four contrasts from a Dixon sequence.

Water Excitation

Water excitation acts to excite water only and not fat. How does that work? Something not often said – the 90° and 180° RFs in any routine sequence have a "transmitted bandwidth"

Water Only: No Fat signal   Fat Only: No Water signal

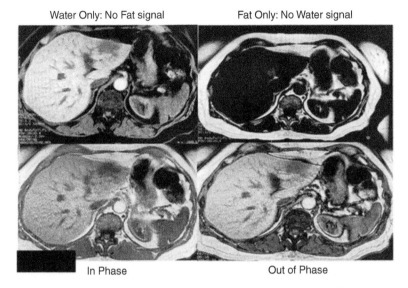

In Phase   Out of Phase

Figure 6.18 The four different contrasts obtained with a Dixon sequence are: Top. Water only and fat only. Bottom. In and out of phase echoes.

Teaching Moment: The "water only" is not "fat-sat," it just looks like it. On the water only, fat is mathematically eliminated. The same is true for the fat only images: Water signal is mathematically taken away. Recall that saturation is to specifically target a specific tissue with an RF pulse to diminish its signal. The water only is often used post gadolinium in the abdomen.

or range of frequencies that excite both water and fat. A water excitation sequence does only that, it excites only water. The 90–180° RFs are tuned to water (fat is excluded from excitation). No transverse NMV for fat develops, meaning no signal. It is basically the opposite of fat-sat where you excite fat first and follow with a 90–180° RF that saturates fat. With water excitation, the 90° and 180° are tuned to water's PF so only water-containing structures give signal. Everybody else sits on the side-lines. You are again taking advantage of the chemical shift between fat and water. If you excite only water, you will only get signal from water (Figures 6.19–6.21).

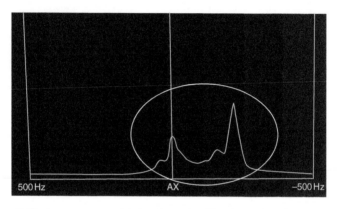

Figure 6.19 A spectrum with both peaks. The RF pulse that caused this spectrum had a wide bandwidth that excited both fat and water (circled: water left, fat right). The separation between the peaks is called "chemical shift."

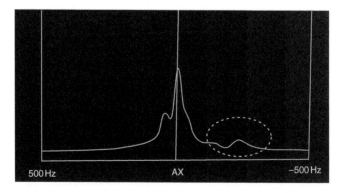

Figure 6.20 In water excitation, the RF has frequencies that only excite water. Fat (circled) is not excited so gives little to no signal.

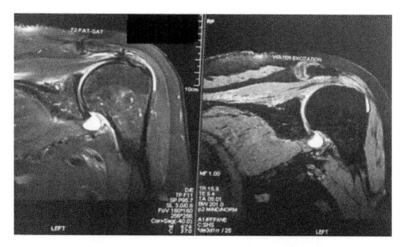

Figure 6.21 T2 fat-sat on the left and water excitation on the right. Both have very similar contrasts. Water excludes fat from the image by NOT exciting it so it gives no signal. We are exploiting the T1 relaxation differences between water and fat. Fat is not allowed to play the game. Remember that **fat-sat** is a saturation technique (chemical saturation) with an RF pulse tuned to the PF of fat. You only see water-containing structures in both fat-sat and water excitation techniques. Water excitation is an easier sequence to do as fat-sat is rife with opportunities to fail or have artifacts. We always do fat-sat because we can fat-sat just about any sequence, but water excitation is not available on all sequences.

Saturation Pulses or Bands

A saturation band is a user-placeable zone of RF that is used to control several artifacts: Gross patient motion (Figure 6.22), pulsatile artifacts, wrap, or aliasing. **A saturation band's RF B/W is wide to excite all the tissue it covers.**

Saturation pulses will increase SAR, and will probably require an increased TR, so longer scan times. Be careful with the T1 contrast with increased TR.

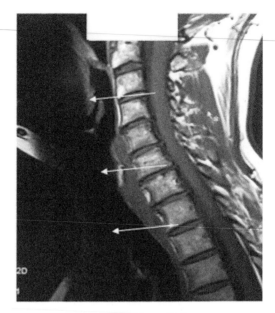

Figure 6.22 An anteriorly placed saturation pulse (arrows). Here it is used to decrease breathing/swallowing motion.

Review: There are two ways to decrease signal from tissues: Suppression and saturation. **IRs** use a tissue's T1 relaxation time and a TI to suppress different tissues.

- *IRs:* **Long TIs** suppress long T1 tissue; **short TIs** suppress short T1 tissue.
- *Saturation:* **Fat-sat** uses RF pulses tuned to the PF of fat to give it three quick 90°s, causing fat-sat. **Water sat** uses the same RF pattern: three quick 90°s suppress H_2O.
- *Dixon* takes away signal mathematically by adding/subtracting the IP and OOP TEs. It is neither a suppression nor a saturation method.
- *Water excitation* shows signal from H_2O only by exciting just water protons. Fat gives no signal as it is not excited.

Subtractions

Subtractions (subs) are very common in contrast MRA and breast and abdominal/pelvic studies. Subtraction images have been around for years. One tissue is digitally subtracted from another. The pre-image set (DRY) is taken away from the post-image set (WET). I like to describe it as: WET–DRY. The purpose of subs is to see only the gadolinium by taking away the background T1 signal. Subs are not really for vividly enhancing lesions, like those in the brain. The brain does not actually enhance.

Subs are most often used in breast and abdomen. The kidney, liver, or breast enhances vividly, as will a lesion. When an organ enhances and a lesion equally enhances, what do you have? **Not much contrast between those tissues**. Subs will take away the kidney/liver/breast, leaving a gadolinium-filled lesion. Ideally:

- The patient has held still and is in the exact same position on the Pre's and the Post's. This way tissues will subtract (cancel each other out). The only difference between them should be gadolinium enhancement.
- The patient ideally needs to have consistent breathing to avoid mis-registration. If breathing is off, a sub is still possible, but the tissues will not subtract correctly, which equals mis-registration. Images of mis-registration are shown in Figures 6.23 and 6.24.

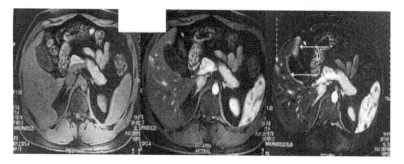

Figure 6.23 Example of a good subtraction with only very slight mis-registration as shown by the light area in proximity to the gallbladder (solid white arrows). Also note how nicely the hemangioma is visualized on the subtraction (dashed arrow).

Pre   Post   Subtraction

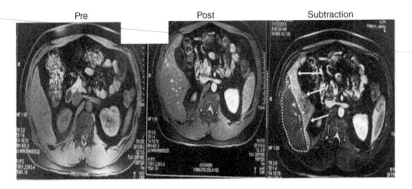

Figure 6.24 Subtraction at mid to lower liver. The patient's respiration was different from pre to post. Note only partial subtraction of the liver. The subtracted area (right image) is within the dotted circle; the un-subtracted area is shown with white arrows. The dotted circle is the same size and shape as the pre-liver. Table positions were the same, but the anatomy was at different positions from pre to post. The same thing happened in the spleen.

Subtractions: Summary: Subtraction is a way to make the gadolinium stand out better. If there is **no** enhancement in a suspected lesion then there is a signal void in the corresponding subtracted area: A dark area – a dark area = dark. Any absorption of the gadolinium by a lesion on the post gadolinium images is seen as increased signal on the subtracted area: Bright – dark = bright.

Considerations to Do Subtractions: The pre/post TR/TE, F/A, FOV, phase FOV, matrix, slice thickness and slice positions must be **exactly** the same.

Why Do Subtractions?: Subs give increased tumor conspicuity. Signal from blood products is removed (hematomas appear as signal voids, aiding in diagnostic differentials). Overall contrast enhancement is increased (Figures 6.25–6.28).

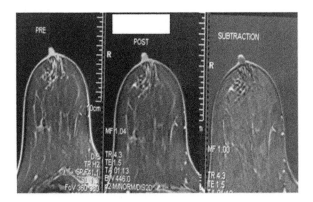

Figure 6.25 Three images of the same breast: Pre, post, and sub. **Note**: The retro-areolar area is bright pre and post but dark on sub: Bright – bright = dark. The lesion is bright on sub: Bright (post) – dark (pre) = bright (just seeing the gadolinium).

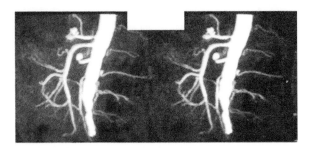

Figure 6.26 Sagittal abdominal MRA. Sub is on the right. Note loss of background signal on subtraction.

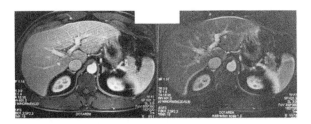

Figure 6.27 Post liver on the left and its sub on the right. Note that paraspinal and subcutaneous tissues are dark on the subtraction. Major vessels in the liver are better seen on the subs because the liver parenchyma is somewhat suppressed by the subtraction process.

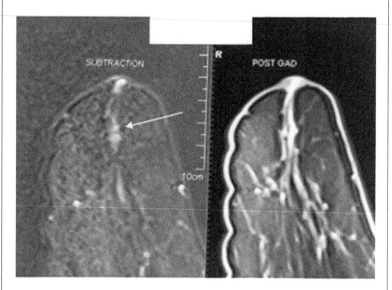

Figure 6.28 Images of breast during biopsy. Note that the retro-areolar area is bright on the sub, demonstrating the lesion to be biopsied.

Another Way to Think of Subtractions

Every tissue has an amount of signal on an image. Let's say the liver on a pre-contrast series has a signal intensity (SI) of 50. On the arterial series with all the gadolinium in the arteries and none in the parenchyma of the liver it also has an SI of 50. The subtraction math is $50 - 50 = 0$, so the liver is very dark on the arterial phase. A 0 SI on the sub, besides being dark, also means **no tissue contrast**. On a venous phase 30 s later, the liver now has an SI of 100 (sub math: $100 - 50 = 50$). The liver is bright, and a slowly enhancing lesion is at, say, 75 ($75 - 50 = 25$) and the lesion is sort of bright against a bright liver; this equals' **contrast**. A third phase with the liver is even brighter at an SI of 150 and now the lesion is at 125, which means the lesion is brighter than in the first phase but not as bright as the liver **so there is still some contrast between them.** The lesion's slow enhancement is a clue as to what it is.

Where is this going? Normal liver/spleen/kidney do the same thing time and again. They are the controls in the MR experiment, with gadolinium as the variable. Pathologies will enhance with different patterns and speeds, and have different amounts of signal. Primary tumors or metastases enhance differently than a haemangioma will. It is the radiologists' job to know the differences, it is our job to show it to them.

Magnetization Transfer

Magnetization transfer (MT) suppresses (just lessens) signal from one tissue in order to see another better. Previously I have talked about making signal suppression where, basically, you did not want to see it all. This is not what MT does; MT just **decreases** the signal of a tissue a little bit. There are two common applications, both in the brain. MT is commonly used in brain MRA's to decrease signal from WM, making vessels in a circle of Willis (COW) MRA appear brighter. The second application, also in the brain, is in post contrast sequences, again to decrease the signal from WM and increase the conspicuity of MS lesions.

Although MT is used on both T1s and MRAs, it actually takes advantage of the T2 relaxation differences between tissues. It works by applying an "off center" or "off resonant" RF pulse to tissues that have very short T2 times. These are the "bound" protons. The RF pulse causes them to be "magnetized," then they transfer this magnetization to another tissue, the "free" protons. These free protons have a longer T2 relaxation time. Think of this transfer of magnetization like ripples in a pond. Drop a pebble in one end the pond and eventually the ripple reaches the other end. Figure 6.29 demonstrates this effect.

The "off center" RF pulse **does not affect** the "free" protons directly (it is not at the PF of water) but instead affects the "bound," which are not seen in routine imaging. **MT will** increase SAR, lengthen the minimum TE (which may require a slightly longer TR), and lengthen scan time (Figure 6.30).

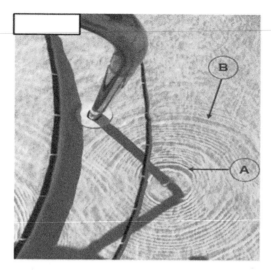

Figure 6.29 I was gently shaking the handrail in a pool. The water acted to magnify the "ripples," pointed out by arrows. This shows how an energy (RF) starts in one location, tissue "A", and transfers to another, tissue "B." Tissue A transfers its magnetization to tissue B, which ultimately gives less signal. Here "B" is less dark, which on an MR image means less signal.

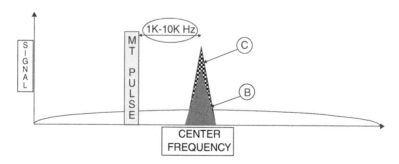

Figure 6.30 Off center RF excites the slice; bound tissues transfer its magnetization to free tissue B also within the same slice. Tissue B gives less signal at TE. C (checkered area) represents the signal that B would have given if it were not for the effects of the MT pulse.

If you are confused by the free and bound protons, off center RF pulse, you are not alone. Let's un-confuse things.

The MT Skinny: First: Think of the MT pulse as nothing more than a preparatory pulse. It is slice selective, meaning it is applied to each slice just like a 90° or 180°. It actually precedes the 90–180° RF PSD (Figure 6.31).

Second: The center frequency (CF) of the MT pulse is not the same as the 90°. It is off the CF by 1000–10,000 Hz so it does not excite the slice for imaging, but selectively saturates hydrogen in bound or restricted tissues like the WM. It is like a fat-sat pulse but for WM. Call it a WM sat pulse if you like.

Third: At TE, the WM is saturated a little bit so, by giving less signal, other tissues like blood vessels and MS plaques are brighter and better seen.

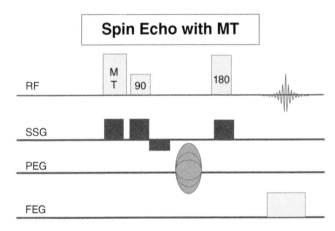

Figure 6.31 A basic SE PSD with an MT pulse preceding the 90°.

IR Prepped Sequences

An IR prepped sequence can be either SE or FSE (both 2D sequences) or, if it is a GRE, 3D. These can have multiple contrast weightings in which a 180° RF pulse or pulses are applied to enhance contrasts between tissues or in some cases to suppress tissues.

If you really think about it, all pulse sequences have three basic components: a prep component, then an acquisition portion, and finally a relaxation or recovery period. Let's break that down a bit. In a simple SE sequence, the "prep" component is the **90–180°** RF pulses, then an Echo is **acquired** and, after the echo, there is time for T1 **relaxation**. What about a basic STIR? The **180–90–180°** RF's constitute the "prep" portion, then the echo is **acquired**, and finally T1 **relaxation**. These three basic occurrences are in all sequences.

IR Prepped Pulses

I shall explain two different kinds of IR prep pulses, called selective or non-selective. It is more correct to think of them as "frequency selective" or "non-frequency selective" RF pulses.

An IR prep pulse is considered "non-selective" when the 180° RF pulse excites **all** the tissue in a slice or slab, whereas a "selective" RF pulse has a particular set of RF frequencies within it targeting a certain tissue. SPAIR or SPIR are examples of selective IR sequences, but fat-sat, while not an inversion pulse, is selective as its RF targets fat. Now, contrast that with the basic STIR and FLAIR sequences which use "non-selective" RF pulses. Recall from earlier in the chapter that SPAIR/SPIR uses a 180° inversion pulse which is specifically tuned with TIs to target fat.

Think back to earlier in this book when I explained the basic SE pulse sequence. If you really think about it, both the 90° (or an excitation pulse) and the 180° RF pulses are "non-selective" RF pulses as they excite/refocus all the tissues in the slice/slab.

The common use of an IR prepped sequence beyond STIR and FLAIR is the 3D IR prepped 3D GRE in the brain to **enhance** GM/WM differentiation on either pre or post gadolinium T1 images. These for example are (vendor specific here) the BRAVO, 3D-TFE, and MP-RAGE. These are commonly used as T1 weighted pre and post contrast pulse sequences. They use a single IR prep pulse to enhance tissue contrast.

Then there is what is called a "double inversion recovery," also used in the brain. It is used to **suppress** two tissues, CSF and WM, thus leaving MS plaques brighter than the adjacent WM. These double IR pulse sequences have two IR pulses, like the name suggests. Double inversion recovery employs a short TI to suppress WM, and a long TI to suppress CSF.

Recall that a short TI suppresses short T1 tissues while a long TI suppresses long T1 relaxing tissues. Also remember that the time between the IR pulse (the 180°) and excitation pulse is the TI. Some vendors also allow for a fat-sat pulse to suppress subcutaneous fat. This makes the sequence rather low SNR as you are suppressing several different tissues and also pretty RF intense with a fat-sat and two different 180° RF pulses.

In the Double IR sequence (used to specifically make blood flow dark) the TIs are adjusted to decrease signal (suppress) from certain tissues.

Figure 6.32 is an example of a double inversion recovery sequence in the brain. Note that the WM is very dark, coming from the short TI, and the CSF is also dark from the long TI.

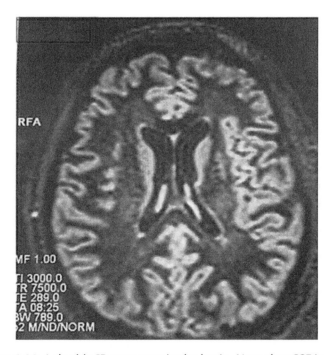

Figure 6.32 A double IR sequence in the brain. Note that CSF is dark from the long TI, and WM is also dark from the short TI. On the sequence, MS plaques are/will be bright as their T1 relaxation time is different from CSF and WM.

Teaching Moment: You will also note that the image in Figure 6.32 is rather low SNR and not really visually pleasing (i.e. not pretty). Remember that images do not have to be "pretty" to be diagnostic. If the images answer the diagnostic question, they are beautiful.

How is an RF Pulse Selective or Non-Selective?

The "selective" or "non-selective" name comes from the transmitter bandwidth. Does the transmitted RF pulse contain a range of frequencies that includes both fat and water, or does it not?

If an RF pulse contains both fat and water frequencies, then it will excite and refocus both of them. That's "non-selective." In SPAIR/SPIR, pulses contain RF that will only excite fat. That is "selective."

The 90° and 180° RF pulses in, say, an SE have both fat and water frequencies: non-selective.

Lastly, fat saturation. The saturation pulses in fat-sat sequences are selective as they contain only the frequencies for fat. They are, however, not inversion pulses as they only flip fat's NMV into the 90° or X/Y.

The drawback of these sequences or methods is an increase in both SAR and scan time. They have extra RF pulses (SAR), and the extra work required for applying the RF and gradients costs time.

Figure 6.33 shows three different RF pulse playouts. The top example is a fat-sat line diagram. The three RFs before the 90° have only frequencies for fat and are "selective," meaning only fat is excited. Fat will give little to no signal at TE.

The middle diagram is the basic STIR/FLAIR. The 180° IR pulse contains both fat and water frequencies so both tissues are inverted. The TI decides which tissue, fat or water, will

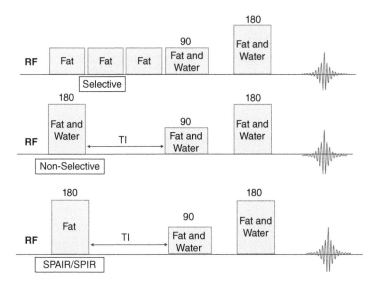

Figure 6.33 Three RF pulse playouts. See text for explanation.

be nulled at TE. Short TIs suppress all short T1 tissue – fat, gadolinium, and proteins – while long TIs suppress long T1 tissues: CSF.

The bottom diagram is, as noted, a SPAIR or SPIR. The inversion pulse is a 180° RF pulse but it has a narrow-transmitted bandwidth of frequencies to only invert fat while not exciting/inverting water and is considered a "selective" inversion pulse. It is a hybrid of sorts: Inversion like a STIR or FLAIR but selective in its tissue to suppress.

Teaching Moment: Speaking of T1 times, as an FYI, urine also has a long T1 time because it is mostly water, like CSF. In real-time everyday scanning you will be using techniques to suppress CFS signal in the brain, not urine in the pelvis. The long T1 time of urine is why you will see "cross-excitation" artifacts in scouts in the bladder (see "Cross-Excitation" in Chapter 12).

Occasionally you may be asked to do something called an MRU (MR urography) where you are specifically using a very heavily T2 weighted sequence to see the renal collecting system, ureters, and bladder. This is your standard MRCP sequence, just centered for imaging the genitourinary system.

Water Excitation Sequences

Water excitation sequences are a fancy way to get signal from water but not fat. It is not a fat-sat technique, but that is the end result: Little to no signal from fat. A water excitation sequence uses a series of partial flip angle RF pulses that excites both water and fat. These RF pulses are timed to ultimately have mostly water in the X/Y plane and not fat in at TE. In this case you could consider it "non-selective" as you are targeting a tissue to be suppressed with a wide transmitted B/W that includes both fat and water frequencies.

Water excitation sequences use a "bi-nominal" (two part) series of partial flip angle RF pulses. The sequence begins with a 22.5°, a short delay, a 45°, another delay, and finishes with another 22.5° RF pulse followed by echo formation.

The short delays between the RF pulses are designed to allow for fat to partially T1 relax, while water will T1 very little during those delays. The end result is that water's NMV is in the X/Y plane or 90° (22.5 + 45 + 22.5 = 90). This pulse scheme and timing results in little to no NMV for fat in the X/Y plane at TE. See Figure 6.21 for a water excitation image in the shoulder.

Notes

7

The Gradient Echo Sequence

Chapter at a Glance

MRI Physics: Tech to Tech Explanations, First Edition. Stephen J. Powers.
© 2021 John Wiley & Sons Ltd. Published 2021 by John Wiley & Sons Ltd.

The other kind of sequence in MRI is the gradient echo. This is referred to in several different ways: gradient recalled echo (GRE), gradient echo (GE), or sometimes T2*. It uses a different mechanism to produce an echo. There is an RF excitation pulse to push the NMV into the X/Y. This is followed by a pair of gradient pulses to de-phase, then re-phase, the protons. An echo results, hence the name gradient echo. GREs can be used to produce any of the three weightings, T1, T2*, and PD. T1 and T2* are the most commonly acquired of the three weightings.

What is a gradient? Any hill or incline is a grade or gradient. You have seen the sign in Figure 7.1 before. It warns trucks to use a low gear as there is a steep hill ahead. In MR, a gradient is a magnetic hill or slope. Chapter 13 explains gradients in more detail.

A gradient pulse can do the same job as an RF pulse to refocus or re-phase the NMV. It cannot, however, excite tissues like RF can, but once excited, gradients can be used to cause an echo.

Figure 7.1 Road sign for a gradient.

Teaching Moment: GRE sequences have less SAR/RF than an SE or TSE sequence. There is only one excitation pulse. They can also have a far shorter TR/TE than an SE as applying a magnetic gradient takes less time than an RF pulse. Also, you do not have to wait half the TE to apply the 180° and half for the echo. That is why GREs are used to do MRAs and not SEs: They have short TEs.

GRE Sequence Structure

Gradient echo sequences have more gradients applied than an SE. Any time you turn on a field gradient, you change the magnetic field and protons de-phase. That is called "phase dispersion," meaning any phase coherence the protons may have had is negatively affected by a gradient being turned on. De-phasing causes a loss of signal.

If one gradient application de-phases the NMV, one can be used to re-phase it. That correction is done with a gradient that is turned on with **equal** strength and **opposite** polarity (Figures 7.2 and 7.3). That is the equivalent to a +90° RF pulse being cancelled out by a -90° RF pulse.

This is the basis for GREs. Flip the NMV with an RF pulse, apply gradient "A" to cause dispersion, follow with gradient "B" to fix it, and an echo results. That echo is called a gradient echo.

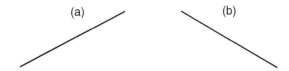

(a)   (b)

Figure 7.2 Gradient A is opposed by an equal and opposite gradient, B. Any effects of gradient A are corrected for by gradient B. **Equal and opposite is key.**

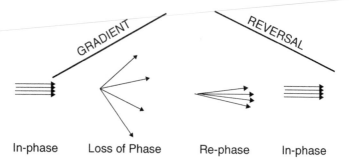

| In-phase | Loss of Phase | Re-phase | In-phase |

Figure 7.3 Visual depiction of a loss of phase caused by a gradient, followed by a gradient reversal for correction.

Phase Dispersion and Gradient Reversal

Which gradient does the refocusing? The FEG causes the echo to form. During a GRE, two different gradients do the job of causing de-phasing and then re-phasing. It is always the SSG and the FEG.

In **all** sequences, the SSG is applied during excitation to locate the slice, but turning on the SSG de-phases things a little so an opposite polarity, SSG, is applied to correct the effects of the first SSG. You will see this in all PSD diagrams. In Figure 7.4, a GRE line diagram (PSD), the FEG is applied twice. First it causes de-phasing #1, and then #2 to re-phase, which ultimately causes echo formation (circled).

Here is the breakdown for Figure 7.4:

RF: The excitation pulse for a slice.
SSG: Slice select gradient: Magnetic field and RF applied.
PEG: Phase encoding gradient. Determines which line of k-space the echo will fill.
FEG: Frequency encoding gradient.
ADC: Analog to digital converter: When you see "ADC" you can think of this as the coil being turned on.

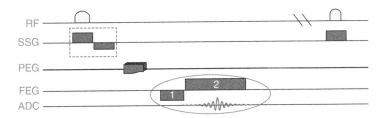

Figure 7.4 The RF and SSG are applied simultaneously with an opposite polarity SSG right after to re-phase the effects of the initial SSG (dashed rectangle). Later on, the FEG is applied, #1, to cause de-phasing, followed by an **equal and opposite** polarity gradient, #2, correcting the effects of the #1, which causes echo formation.

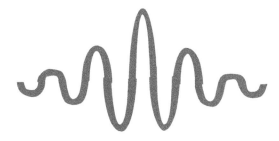

Figure 7.5 Analog wave form.

Analog to Digital Converter (ADC)

The echo is actually an oscillating wave. That is because the NMV is pointing at the coil, then is not, then is, then is not, and so on. This wave form is considered an **analog** signal (Figure 7.5).

Fourier transform cannot work on a wave form; it needs numbers, so there is a device called an ADC. It **converts analog** signals into numbers or **digits**, hence **analog to digital converter**.

GRE Sequence Image Weighting

- GREs are very versatile sequences.
- They have a great number of uses, from MRA to musculoskeletal to neurology.

- GREs can be weighted T1, T2 (actually T2*) and PD.
- GREs can be 2D and 3D.

Teaching Moment: Calling a GRE T2 weighted is not exactly correct. It cannot be T2 weighted. T2 comes from an SE. A GRE can look T2 like with bright fluid but a GRE's contrast comes from magnetic susceptibilities and local and main magnetic field inhomogeneities (the stuff the 180° cleans up for).

Many techs struggle with GREs in general because there are variations in weighting that are not exactly straightforward.

Know that there are two kinds of GREs: **Standard and steady state (SS)**. **Standard** has a longish TR and TE and a shallow F/A. These are mostly used in the brain to look for hemorrhage, or axials in the cervical spine. **SS** has two different kinds: **Coherent and incoherent**. SS typically has a very short TR/TE and can have T1 or T2 looking contrasts. There is more on the SS to come. I wanted to get this out there before the confusion starts.

There is a another parameter in GREs besides TR and TE: the F/A. The F/A is how far the B_0 NMV is "Flipped" into the Transverse or X/Y plane. TR does little to the weighting as compared to its effects in SE. TE is still for "T2" weighting. The **F/A** has a big effect on image contrast. When you hear "GRE," the first thing you should think of is: What is the F/A? In SE the F/A is assumed to be 90° unless otherwise stated.

Most techs struggle with GRE weighting. For me, at first, it was brute memorization with no clue of what the TR, TE, F/A did. Then a physicist gave me this nugget. He called it a "teaching moment" and that is why I use the term.

Teaching Moment: Consider all GREs T2 until you make them T1 weighted.
Here is how GREs can be made T1:

- Keep the TE short to minimize T2 (just like in SE).
- Think of the F/A as your T1. To increase T1 contrast, increase the F/A. All factors being the same, a 60° F/A has more T1 than a 25°. If you put T1 contrast in with a higher F/A, expect to get T1 back in your echo.

A short TE = less T2, and a large F/A = more T1. In the previously explained weighting triangle, T1 will be on top.

How does the **F/A** contribute to T1 contrast? Think back to SE. The F/A is assumed to be 90° so the NMV has a lot of "T1'ing" to do going to B_0 vs. a 25° F/A. Which one has more T1'ing to do? The answer is 90°. The NMV has more ground to cover from 90° than it does from 25°.

TR in GRE has less to do with image contrast than it does in an SE sequence. TR's contributions or effects in GREs are:

- It allows more slices (increased scan coverage).
- It has decreased saturation effects as the protons have time to "Stand-up". A 300 ms TR vs. an 800 ms TR allows more time T1 relaxation to occur so less chance of saturation (Figure 7.6).

The **TE** still controls T2 contrast; however, the TE times do decrease. A 90 ms TE in GRE is very long and will have very little SNR but would be just fine in SE land. A long TE in GRE is in the 25–35 ms range. Short TEs would be about 3–7 ms. That said, with all factors remaining the same, an SE will have a higher SNR than a GRE. That is because of the 180° in SE.

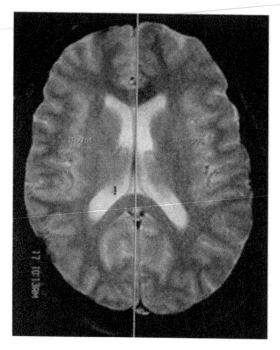

Figure 7.6 Split screen, same slice, same patient shows two different axials with different TRs. The left was scanned at 760 ms, the right at 1200 ms. The most obvious difference is that WM on the right is darker compared to the left. Scan time was almost twice as long. TR in GRE land has less to do with image contrast than it does in an SE.

Let's introduce a new concept here: A GRE is often called a **T2* (T2 star).**

Where does the "star" come from? Know that there are two forms of T2 relaxation. They happen simultaneously and for different reasons. Hear GRE, think T2*; hear T2*, think GRE. The * denotes that the echo came from a gradient reversal (refocusing) not RF refocusing.

Two Different Kinds of T2 Relaxation

True T2 or spin-spin is basically protons that leave the transverse plane due to field small field inhomogeneities and spin-spin interactions. Spin-spin interactions are the protons acting like bumper cars. They crash into each other and leave the X/Y plane. They are gone and you do not get them back until the next TR. The 180° in a SE does not bring them back into alignment.

The other "T2" relaxation is called **T2***. T2* happens because of field inhomogeneities and chemical shifts. **The protons de-phase but they stay in the X/Y plane.** A 180° will correct or re-phase the T2* de-phasing. **Re-phasing them with RF causes an echo called a "spin echo."** SE echoes can be T1, T2, or PD weighted.

In a GRE, the same true T2 and T2* relaxations happen but the **gradient reversal** (not RF) used to produce the echo does not correct for the de-phasing like a 180°. The resultant echo is a **T2***. **T2* echoes can be T1, T2, or PD weighted.**

SE sequences are considered to be the "gold standard" in MRI. GRE images can look T2 with bright fluid but it is not the same process as in an SE. You could say it is "T2 like." Speaking of bright fluid, as an FYI, all sequences that have bright fluid are not necessarily T2 weighted.

Another question I have heard is: How do you visually identify FSE vs. GRE without knowing the scan parameters?

- Look at the images for overall SNR; it is lower on GRE.
- Look for susceptibility artifacts at air/tissue interfaces. GRE will have some warping at those interfaces.

The GRE Weighting Triangle

Remember: Think of F/A as T1 contrast being put into the image. The higher the F/A, the more T1 relaxing the NMV has to do to go back to longitudinal (B_0), so this will be seen in the image (Figures 7.7 and 7.8).

Let's Use What We Already Know:

- Old school SE PD has a short TE to decrease T2, and long TR to decrease T1. In GRE, a short TE (5–7 ms) will decrease T2*.
- Use of a shallow F/A (5–15°) also lessens T1.
- Minimize T1 and minimize T2*: **PD wins**.
- You may be using PD GREs and not even know it.

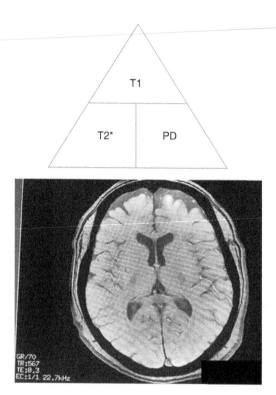

Figure 7.7 Using a higher F/A (50–90°), expect more T1 contrast; short TEs let less T2* happen. Add T1 and minimize T2*: T1 wins.

For Figures 7.8 and 7.9 let's compare the PD to T2* images:

- Both have bright fluid.
- T2*: Figure 7.8 CSF is brighter with good GM/WM contrast.
- PD: Figure 7.9 has brighter fat with better GM/WM differentiation.

Both will work for hemorrhage but the T2* (Figure 7.8) would be my choice to see hemorrhage. It has a longer TE to take advantage of the extra de-phasing.

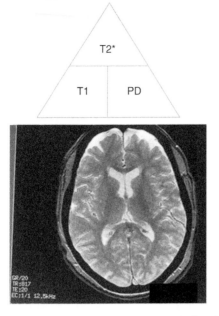

Figure 7.8 A longer TE to more T2* contrast and a shallow/low F/A to decrease T1 contrast: T2* wins. CSF is brighter with good GM/WM contrast.

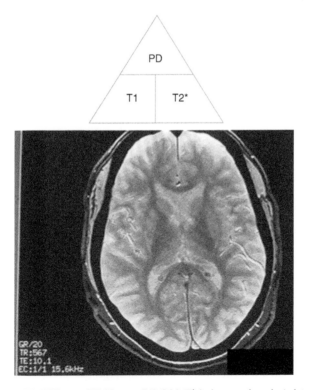

Figure 7.9 TR 567 ms, TE 10 ms, F/A 20°. This image has brighter fat, and better GM/WM differentiation.

GRE and SE Differences

The major difference between GRE and SE is the way the echo is produced. The 180° refocusing pulse in SE is the key. What the 180° does is clean up or help decrease the effects of de-phasing caused by multiple things, local and main magnetic field inhomogeneities and magnetic susceptibilities "The Big Three").

What causes these inhomogeneities/susceptibilities?

- In the brain, metal from dental work, surgery, air in the sinuses, and what has already been mentioned, blood.
- Blood has hemoglobin, hemoglobin contains iron. Iron is a metal. Metal adversely affects the local magnetic field homogeneity, causing an area of loss of signal (Figure 7.10). Arrows point to areas of inhomogeneity on the left, cleaned up on the right by the series of 180°s in an FSE.

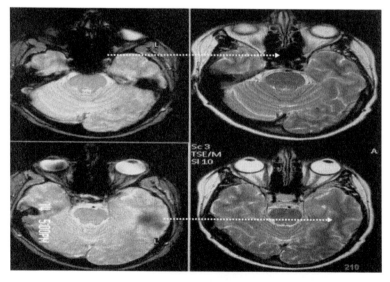

Figure 7.10 Same patient, same slices in GRE on the left and FSE on the right. Note how the inhomogeneity artifact from the air in the paranasal and petrous ridges is corrected for by the echo train in the FSE.

Metal Artifact on a TSE and GRE

See Figure 7.11.

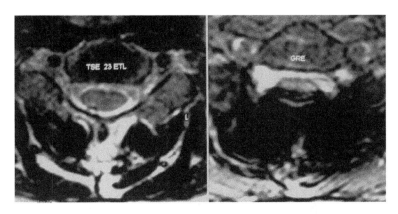

Figure 7.11 On the left is an FSE with ETL of 23, and on the right is a GRE. Note the amount of metal artifact reduction on the FSE with the many 180°s vs. the GRE with none. Same patient, same slice.

Different Gradient Echo Types

So far all I have done is describe the basic GRE sequence. There are actually two other variations or types of GRE. This section will help you understand the differences between them and their uses. These two types or variations are **steady state and spoiled.** Lots of different names get used describing/naming these sequences. If you are confused, you are not alone. All vendors have their own names for them.

Recall I said that GREs can have very short TRs and TEs. Sometimes the TR is shorter than both the T1 and T2 times of tissues. What this means is that, after the TE, there is left-over transverse NMV. With a very short TR, the leftovers do not have enough time to T1 or T2 relax before the next excitation. Something needs to get done with the leftovers.

GRE's leftovers:

The leftovers are called a residual NMV. The residual NMV is/are the long T1 and T2 relaxing tissues. This is where the steady state or spoiled terminology comes in. If the NMV is to be thrown away it is called spoiled; if kept for use by the next TR it is called steady state.

Spoiled and steady state are general terms used to describe what is going to happen to those leftovers.

Spoiled GRE

Let's start with **spoiled** as it is the easiest to understand. Spoiling means the leftovers are forced to go away, de-phased, or crushed. You have probably heard or used the term **SPGR** (spoiled gradient recalled echo). As soon as you hear the term **spoiled, think a T1 weighted GRE**. These sequences are often used pre and post gadolinium. These are your BRAVOs, MP-RAGE, LAVA, VIBE, VIBRANT, THRIVE, etc. There are many names but all are basically the same sequence: SPGRs. These are also often, but not necessarily, scanned with fat-sat.

An Easy Trick: If you are having trouble getting a T1 fat-sat either pre or post gadolinium, on an off-center FOV, try T1 weighted SPGRs out of your 3D Abdomen sequences. Adjust the FOV to an appropriate size, and the other scan parameters to maintain resolution and SNR. Remember, these are GREs and do not like metal or other causes of field inhomogeneity, but it is worth a shot. You might be pleasantly surprised. I like to say, "If you don't swing, you don't hit anything."

Another new term needs to be introduced here: **Incoherent**. Incoherent and spoiled mean the same thing. Saying spoiled is easier than incoherent. To say a GRE sequence is "incoherent" means it is spoiled. So, how is a sequence "spoiled"? It can be spoiled in one of two ways: An RF pulse or a gradient pulse can be used (Figure 7.12). It does not force the NMV to T1 relax like in driven equilibrium. It just scrambles the leftovers, making them unable to give signal. So, if you make the T2 go away, have a higher F/A and short TE, T1 contrast will dominate. Bingo, SPGR = T1.

Steady State GRE

Now for the steady state version of GRE. Again, the TR is very short so little to no T1 or T2 relaxation gets to occur. This very short TR leaves a residual transverse NMV. In the steady state GRE, you want to keep that NMV to be used for the next TR. This residual NMV will, over a short period of time, start to de-phase.

If spoiled GREs are called incoherent, then, guess what, non-spoiled or **steady state** GREs are **coherent**. Vendor specific names are FIESTA, CISS, FISP, and Balanced FFE. The residual

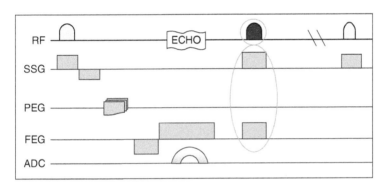

Figure 7.12 An SPGR PSD with the spoiler pulses circled.

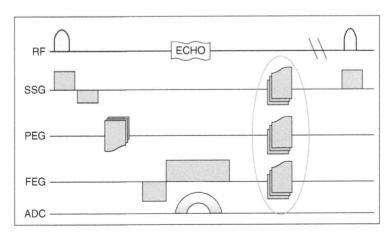

Figure 7.13 A steady state GRE PSD with the re-winding a.k.a. re-phasing gradients circled.

Net Transverse Magnetization (the leftover NMV after the echo) will be re-phased by gradient pulses in all three directions. See Figure 7.13. You are keeping them "steady" over and over again, so they are said to be or described as being in a "steady state."

- It takes a couple of TRs to reach the steady state.
- The NMV spins are reused during the next TR.
- The image contrast is a combination of T1 and T2.
- The image is a compilation of TR, F/A, and T1 /T2 of tissues.
- These SS-GREs typically have bright fluid **but** are not T2 weighted. **The three "Fs" are bright: Fat, fluid, and flow.**

Teaching Moment: Figure 7.14 images show bright fluid (but not T2 weighted), bright fat (but not T1 weighted), and bright flow (but it is not MRA). These sequences are not used for pathology, just anatomy as they are **not T2 weighted.**

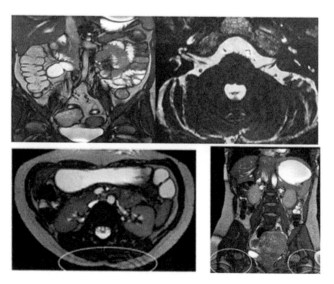

Figure 7.14 Note that the three Fs are bright: Fat, fluid, and flow. Having TRs as short as possible (<4 ms) brightens up the flow and decreases moiré artifact (circled).

Pros and Cons of SS-GREs include:

- High CNR and SNR: Pro.
- Motion insensitivity due to the presence of balanced gradients in all three directions: Pro.
- Can be used for high resolution anatomy or for cardiac, fetal, or gastric motility: Pro.
- Artifact prone: Con. If TR is too long, and if fat-sat'd they like to drift off resonance, especially if off center FOVs are used, so "shim baby, shim."
- Even though these are GRE based, the combination of the very short TR and higher F/A's SNR is rather good: Pro.

In and Out of Phase TEs

Both fat and water T1 and T2 relax at different rates. We can take advantage of these different T2 relaxation rates by acquiring at TEs when fat and water are both pointing in the same direction (in-phase, IP) or when they are pointing in opposite directions (out of phase, or just plain OOP). An out of phase TE is sometimes called an "opposed phase TE" or "phase shift image."

What is really happening? When fat and H_2O are both in the same pixel, they will either "add" to each other (brighter) **in phase**, or they will cancel each other (darker) **out of phase** (Figure 7.15).

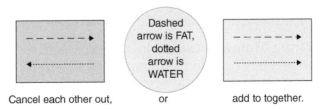

Cancel each other out,   or   add to together.

Figure 7.15 A representation of two different pixels and the vectors present at the time of the echo. The left pixel, with opposing vectors, will be darker compared to the right pixel as the vectors cancel each other out instead of contributing to the overall signal.

You can **only** get IP/OOP images with GREs. Even if you run an SE and acquire the TE at an IP or OOP TE you will not see the out of phase effect. Why? Because the 180° in an SE sequence puts the protons in phase at TE. **You would never get the OOP effect ever.** GREs do not have 180°s.

OK, where do those TE numbers come from? The equation is in the section "In and Out of Phase TEs" in Chapter 14. This equation is seldom mentioned.

The In Phase TE

1/(3.5 ppm × PF) × 1000 = first IP TE. So, 3.5 ppm × 63.86 = 223.51.

Then: 1/223.51 = 0.00446.

Next: 0.00446 × 1000 = 4.46 ms is the first IP TE.

The Out of Phase TE

Take the first IP TE and divide it by 2, then add the IP TE.

4.46/2 = 2.23.

2.23 + 4.46 = 6.69 ms.

Years ago, gradient hardware and software were not as advanced as they are today. This fact pushed the first OOP TE you could acquire out to 6.6 ms. With improvements to scanner technology, the first acquirable OOP TE is 2.2 at 1.5 T.

Teaching Moment: On an IP/OOP sequence, the OOP TE should be acquired first because: (i) shorter TEs will always increase the SNR; and (ii) lengthening the TEs will require a longer TR and may take you out of reasonable breath-hold times. For example: TEs of 4.4 and 6.6 ms will need a longer TR than TEs of 2.2 and 4.4 ms.

In Phase/Out of Phase at 1.5 T

As If You Are Looking Up the Bore at an Axial Slice

Figure 7.16 shows the progression in ms for IP-OOP TEs. At 3 T it is 1.1 ms OOP, 2.2 ms IP, 3.3 ms OOP because the rate of T2 relaxation speeds up at 3 T thus shorter IP-OOP TEs.

Teaching Moment: Some sites are using IP-OOP TE sequences to help differentiate vertebral compression fractures from pathological fractures due to metastases. Benign vertebral fractures will contain fatty marrow (dark on OOP) while a malignancy replaces normal marrow so is bright on OOP.

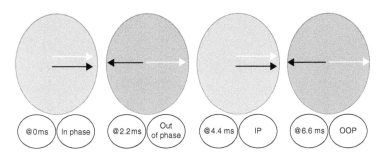

Figure 7.16 The progression in ms for IP/OOP TEs.

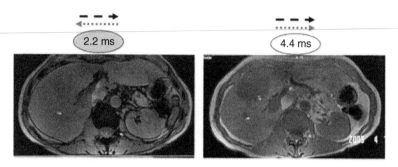

Figure 7.17 OOP and IP axials in the abdomen. Note the decrease in signal of fat, especially in the vertebral body.

In Figure 7.17, OOP is on the left, IP on the right. Note the IP image, it is a T1 weighted image. Also note the signal intensity of fat on the OOP. It is darker than you might expect when you compare it to the IP.

Notes

8

Gradient Echo Magnetic Resonance Angiography

Chapter at a Glance

MRI Physics: Tech to Tech Explanations, First Edition. Stephen J. Powers.
© 2021 John Wiley & Sons Ltd. Published 2021 by John Wiley & Sons Ltd.

RA pulse sequences have been a staple in MRI for years. All MRA sequences are GREs that use a very short TR and TE. The flip angles used vary on whether it is a 2D or 3D sequence. The first and oldest term used to describe a non-contrast MRA was **Time of flight** (TOF). In a TOF MRA, you are imaging in a shorter **time** than blood can **fly** out of the slice. Blood "flies" in to the slice, gets excited, gives off its signal, and flies out. Fresh unexcited blood replaces it, gets excited, gives its signal, and flies out. This results in bright vessels and dark background tissue. The background tissue being dark is the result of the TR/TE being shorter than the T1/T2 of the tissue. The stationary background tissue quickly becomes saturated from repeated RFs being applied very rapidly. This is because of the very short TRs used in MRAs. Short TRs do not let the stationary tissue T1 relax so it quickly ceases to give much signal. The saturated background is a very good thing. A bright vessel in a dark background is **contrast**.

An alternate term for TOF is **flow related enhancement** (FRE). TOF and FRE are both the same thing. FRE means the vessels are enhanced, which is related to blood flowing through them.

Time of Flight MRA

Understanding the flowing blood vs. stationary tissue concept in TOF MRA is huge. Non-saturated spins are entering the imaging slice or volume, getting excited, giving off their signal, and moving on. Flowing blood will be bright against the dark background tissue. That is contrast, and **contrast in MRA is vital**. We are not talking intravenous (IV) contrast, but image contrast.

Blood Flow Types

Before I get into the golden rules of how to do TOF MRAs, let's cover the different types of blood flow that occur in a blood vessel. While an MRA is typically a quick, cheap, and easy way to image blood vessels it is not without its limitations. The biggest limitation is that it "over-estimates" a stenosis. This means a small stenosis can be seen as bigger than it really is. In Figure 8.1, the true stenosis is the black ovals but, because of the flow dynamics (vortex flow) causing loss of signal, a small stenosis is seen on an MRA as larger (dashed lines).

Figure 8.1 shows the four different flow types.

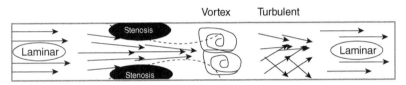

Figure 8.1 TOF MRAs tend to overestimate a stenosis (dashed lines).
Laminar Flow: Normal flow, inner portion moves slightly faster than those close to the vessel walls.
Vortex Flow: Swirling, completely out of phase.
Turbulent Flow: Protons starting to return back to a laminar flow pattern.
Stagnant Flow: Very slow, barely moving.

Table 8.1 describes what the flow types look like.

Table 8.1 What the different flow types look like.

	MRI	MRA
Laminar (plug) flow	Dark	Bright
Vortex flow	Dark	Dark
Turbulent flow	Dark	Dark
Stagnant flow	Bright-ish	Dark

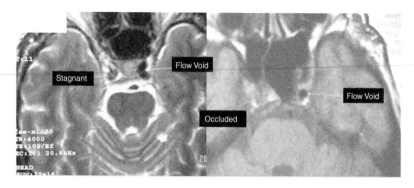

Figure 8.2 SE images. On the left, blood is giving off a little signal as it got the 90° and has not totally exited the slice before TE; some signal is seen. The opposite carotid shows a "flow void." Blood has left the slice. On the right, the carotid siphon is occluded and gives signal as the blood is not moving at all. It acts like stationary tissue. **On MRA it is dark because the short TR/TE causes saturation of very slow flow.**

- *Laminar flow.* **This is dark on SE MRI** as the blood has moved out of the slice between the 90° and the TE. Un-excited blood is in the slice at the TE. Larger vessels are dark/black. This is often called "flow void". Radiologists look for "flow voids" in the major vessels in the brain and will often comment on them (see Figure 8.2 for examples).
- *Vortex and turbulent flow.* Little to no NMV is pointing at the coil, and **no signal is generated for either MRI or MRA.**
- *Stagnant flow.* Signal intensity is a **little bright or grey on MRI**, so this is not quite flow void and not MRA bright either.

Note on the Term "Flow Void": Many radiologists use **"flow void"** to mean a loss of signal in a vessel due to flow-ing blood. "Flow void," while widely used, could be misin-terpreted as having no flow. The term **"High Velocity Signal Loss" (HVSL)** is more accurate to describe **flow in a vessel.** HVSL means the blood has moved out of the slice being imaged and was replaced by **un-excited blood that gives no signal**. HVSL is really the opposite of TOF. HVSL applies to sequences with long TR/TEs.

TOF Angiography: Two Golden Rules

There are a couple of rules that you need to know in order to get the best image quality on your TOF MRAs/MRV's. The first one involves an IV contrast injection and the second one is how to position your slices.

1. TOF MRA or MRV **must** be done **before** any IV contrast injection. Why? TOF MRA is dependent on the T1 relaxation time of blood.
   - Gadolinium shortens the T1 of blood to a point where a saturation pulse becomes ineffective. This means the gadolinium allows blood to T1 relax within the TR period and be able to give off signal at TE. Veins will end up being as bright as arteries despite saturation (sat) pulses.
   - If the patient has already had a gadolinium injection, bring them back tomorrow. A TOF MRA post injection would be a waste of time.
2. Ideally, the TOF MRA slices or slab should be placed orthogonal (at a right angle (90°) to the vessel) to avoid in-plane saturation. In-plane saturation comes from the blood being in the slice or slab too long so it has received many RF pulses and saturates just like the stationary background tissue.

Types of MRA Sequences

There are three different MRA sequences: 2D or 3D TOF; CE-MRA; and phase contrast. A general rule is: **2D TOF** MRA sequences are for **slower flow**, while **3D TOF** is better for **fast flow**. Ideally you want the blood to be in the imaging slab/slice for the shortest time possible (as few RFs as possible). So, if you need an MRV in a leg or arm, go 2D TOF, not 3D. 2D has thin slices (2–4 mm) vs. 3D (a 25–35 mm thick slab). Blood gets through 3 mm slices faster than 30mm thick slabs. You will not get in-plane saturation. 2D can be used on fast and slow flows; 3D does fast flow better than slow flow.

TOF Concept in MRA versus MRV

Arteries and veins have different flow rates but there is always flow in both directions. An MRA/V acquisition can demonstrate either side of the vascular tree by the placement of a sat pulse, placing the sat pulse on the side you do not want to see. You are making it so the unwanted side gets hit with RF before it even enters the imaging volume. It carries this RF with it, gets hit with another RF pulse (RF pulses added), and is saturated at TE (Figures 8.3–8.5).

You also need to consider whether imaging is being done above or below the heart. This will change on which side the sat pulse is placed.

Author's note: I have/make the sat band thicker and closer to the ROI than the system's default for better saturation, especially when saturating the arterial side. Reason, arterial blood flows faster, so fresh spins replace saturated spins sooner.

2D versus 3D

The majority of sequences that are run in MR are "**2D**," meaning the Fourier transform (FT) works on the **phase** and **frequency** encoded data. Two directions = 2D. There are also 3D sequences. In a 3D sequence, the SSG is applied with different amplitudes,

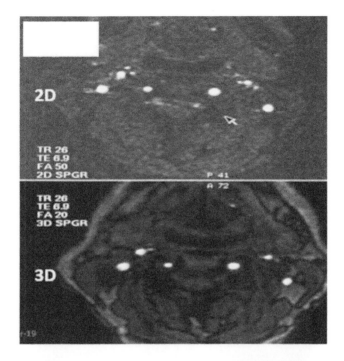

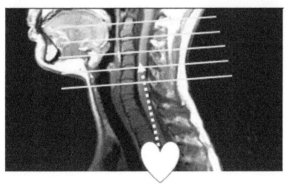

Figure 8.3 Top, middle. The stationary tissue is darker than the flowing blood in the vessels. These are carotid MRA raw data images with the saturation pulse placed superior to the stacks to saturate venous flow entering the slice. Bottom: Placement of a saturation pulse to cancel signal from the venous side of the circulatory tree. Carotid flow is shown by the dotted arrow. Venous flow would of course be in the opposite direction, causing it to be saturated by RF from the saturation pulse, and a second RF from the imaging slice.

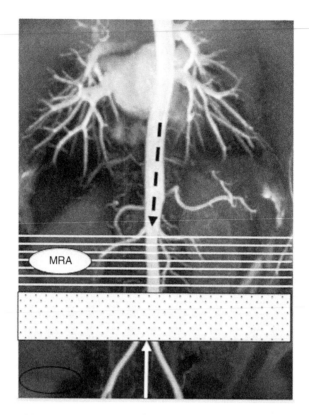

Figure 8.4 Venous sat = MRA. The figure shows venous blood (solid arrow) having to travel through the saturation band, causing it to give no signal from veins, which equals a **2D MRA data set. Am I imaging above or below the heart? That will change which side of the stack you place your sat pulse.**

like the PEG in 2D. This varied amplitude SSG "partitions" the volume into slices (slices within the slice, if you like). When the FT calculates three directions – **slice, phase, and frequency** – it is called a 3D (Figure 8.6; note: circled are SSG, phase, and frequency). Both SSG and PEG are varied amplitudes. This gives the FT three directions to calculate, not just two.

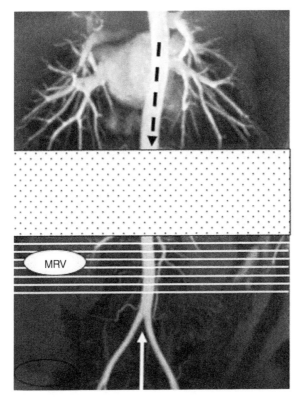

Figure 8.5 Arterial sat = MRV. This figure shows arterial blood (dashed arrow) running through a saturation band, causing no signal from arteries, equalling a **2D MRV data set.**

2D TOF MRAs

2D TOFs are easy to do and reliable, but a drawback is the "stepping" artifact. It is what they do, unfortunately. The stepping in 2Ds is inherent as the sequence is a "sequential" acquisition. That means all the data is acquired from slice 1 before moving on to acquire slice 2, then all of 2, then move on to 3, then 4. See a pattern?

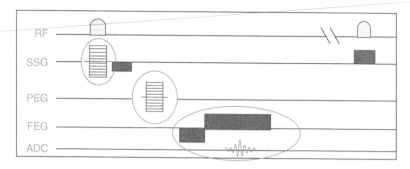

Figure 8.6 A 3D GRE PSD. SSG is varied in amplitude, making the third dimension. Phase PEG and FEG are the other two. All three are circled.

If the patient is moving, the anatomy is in a different position A/P, as seen in Figure 8.7. The vessel does not match up from slice to slice, thus the "stepping".

How can stepping be reduced?

- One way is to scan with slices overlapping by about 20–25%. This will increase scan time as you need more slices for the same coverage with an overlap vs. no overlap.
- Pulse or cardiac gate. These options work well but with set up time and being heart rate dependent can make the sequence rather long.
- IV contrast is also an option. This is covered in Chapter 9 along with k-space.

3D TOF MRAs

A 3D sequence has all the same anatomy as a 2D – RF excitation, slice, phase, and frequency encoding – but one extra, slice select gradient application. That is what makes it a 3D. All things being the same, compared to a 2D, a 3D sequence has higher SNR and higher resolution because of thin slices and a higher matrix.

In a 3D sequence (Figure 8.8), multiplanar reformatting is possible in addition to the ability to cut out the

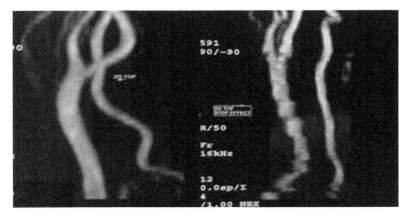

Figure 8.7 The image on the right shows the "stepping" artifact from the patient moving (breathing heavily) in between slices. What has happened is that the anatomy moved within the slice in between slices. While the step artifact is not pretty to look at, all hope is not lost. Radiologists read from the raw data images more than the MIP'd (cut-out) images.

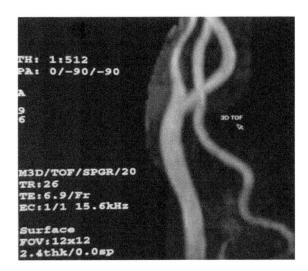

Figure 8.8 A single slab 3D with an inferior to superior ramp pulse (ramp pulses will be explained shortly). Stepping is possible with multi-slab 3D acquisitions for the same reason as in 2D: Patient moves in between slabs.

background tissue for MRAs. 2D sequences are not as good for reformatting as many of them have a gap between slices, but overlapping a 2D MRA sequence will effectively make it into a sort of 3D. These overlapping 2Ds can be reformatted rather well.

In-Plane Saturation

If blood is in a slice/slab too long, it will receive multiple RF pulses and become saturated. This is worse with 3D slabs as they are thicker than 2D slices. There just is not enough time to T1 relax or move out of the slab.

Reasons why blood is in the slab too long:

- When the vessels run **parallel** with the imaging slice or slab, blood, like the stationary tissue, receives multiple RFs and signal in the vessel drops/fades. In Figure 8.9 (in-plane saturation) the vessel runs parallel to the slices (circled).
- The main idea of TOF MRA is for blood to enter the slice/ slab, be excited, give signal, and move on. Even with proper positioning of the slices, in-plane saturation can happen based on patient anatomy (Figure 8.9).

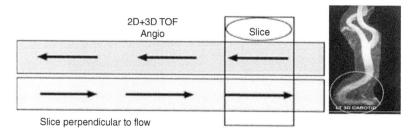

Figure 8.9 The ideal angle (90° or perpendicular) of slice/slab position to flow/vessel for either 2D or 3D TOF.

In-Plane Saturation Avoidance

There are a couple of ways to minimize the effects of in-plane saturation along with proper positioning of the slab.

One is a technique called **MOTSA** (**m**ultiple **o**verlapping **t**hin **s**ection **a**ngiography), which is described next. The other option is called ramped RF, or TONE (tilted optimized non-saturated excitation).

Both of these techniques are often used together and with proper positioning should greatly lessen the in-plane saturation effect. Combined, both work very well but still may not resolve in-plane saturation completely.

MOTSA

As previously stated, if blood flow is in a slab too long, in-plane saturation is possible. A thinner slab lessens the chance of saturation but also affects how much anatomy you can cover. The solution is to scan with several (**multiple**) slabs, to increase coverage, that **overlap** and are **thinner** slabs (sections) for less chance of saturation. The overlap is critical in any kind of imaging, especially angiography, as you do not want to miss any tissue. A general rule to overcome the "stepping" you see as in 2D TOF is an overlap of 20–25% of the 3D slabs (bottom images, Figure 8.10).

Ramped RF Pulse

A "ramped" RF pulse means that the F/A in a slab to be imaged is varied to get the highest contrast possible out of the vessels and background tissue (Figure 8.11). Normally an RF pulse has a "constant" F/A (in SE it is a 90°). A ramped RF pulse is a different kind of RF pulse whose F/A changes as a function of its position. What that means is: A lower F/A is used at the beginning (bottom or foot end) of the slab and is increased towards the head (or top). That is because flowing blood loses signal the higher it is in the slab. A higher F/A will increase the saturation

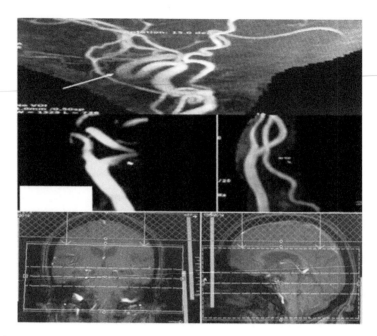

Figure 8.10 Note the carotid, middle right, has uniform signal through the entire length of the vessel. On the left, the vessel makes a turn and fades. Bottom. Coronal and sagittal images demonstrate three thin-section overlapping slabs.

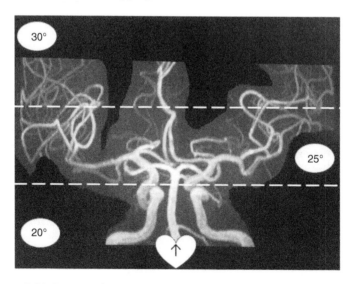

Figure 8.11 A ramped RF increases the F/A in the slab to counter blood saturation. Here ramping is I/S (inferior to superior). For the first third of the slab, F/A is 20°. For the next third, F/A is 25°. The top gets an F/A of 30°. Ramp pulse is applied in the direction of flow you want to see. Ramp direction can be reversed if needed for different flow direction.

of the background tissue, making blood vessels look brighter. Each of the different vendors have its own name and twist on the technique: Philips = Tone Pulse; GE = Ramped; Siemens = T.O.N.E.; Hitachi = SSP Sloped Slab Profile.

Magnetization Transfer (MT)

MT is a tissue suppression technique used in brain MRA and some gadolinium brain scans (for MS).

It is an RF pulse that is absorbed by one tissue, and passed on in turn by that tissue (transferred) to another. It is a WM suppression technique (a mild signal suppression).

It is based on the **T2** relaxation differences of tissues (water vs. proteins) even though it is used on T1 weighted images.

Think of an MT pulse as a "mini sat pulse" to suppress a specific tissue (WM). The MT pulse is applied off the center frequency of H_2O so proteins get excited, not H_2O. The magnetization "ripples" over to water protons (the WM). Proteins give up (transfer) their magnetization to the H_2O, hence magnetization transfer. The results are that at the TE, WM is mildly darker, making gadolinium or flowing blood appear brighter. Gadolinium is not affected by the MT pulse because proteins and gadolinium do not have the same PF.

MT Drawbacks

- The TRs and TEs are likely to increase, which will increase the scan time.
- MT is not able to be used on FSE/TSE sequences; SE only.
- MT is an RF pulse that can affect SAR. This may be an issue on pediatric or newborn imaging. Pediatric patients are not well myelinated so using an RF pulse to suppress something that is not there makes no sense.

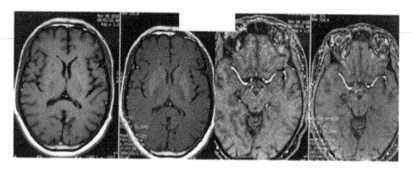

Figure 8.12 Left. T1 axial imaging of the brain with and without MT. Right. 3D MRA images also with and without MT. Same slices, same patient. MT images on the right are "flat" T1 contrast wise.

- MT has a rather limited range of uses, only on neurology (brain) applications, where it is used to see very early MS plaques.
- Less GM/WM differentiation (Figure 8.12).

Teaching Moment: Yes, the image on the right in Figure 8.12 is flat (it lacks GM/WM contrast) but that is OK. If it answers the clinical question, it is a beautiful image. Images do not need to be pretty to be diagnostic.

2D vs. 3D: Pros, Cons and FYIs:

- 2D is better for slower flow, and has better anatomical coverage.
- Due to its thinner slices, 3D has higher resolution.
- 3Ds in general have higher SNR compared to a similar 2D sequence. That is because signal is based on

the 3D volume (20–120 mm thick) vs. a 2D with slice thicknesses of 2–6 mm.

- The higher SNR of 3Ds allows for even higher scan matrices, giving even higher resolution. SNR in 3D increases with an increased number of partitions.
- 3Ds can be easily multiplanar reconstructed, meaning an axial 3D slab can be reconstructed into coronals or sagittals. A 2D set of slices will not look very good.

Options for Better MRAs

- The first thing to use is flow compensation (flow comp). It makes flow bright, which is the reason for an MRA in the first place.
  That is worth the extra TR.
- Try an out of phase TE. An OOP TE can further suppress background tissue (fat gets a little darker).
- OOP at 1.5 T is either 2.2 or 6.6 ms. A 6.6 ms TE may be too long for some radiologists. The longer TE means more de-phasing and loss of signal.
- At 3 T: 1.1 and 3.3 ms. If you can get the first OOP phase TE, great, the second TE is still pretty short.
- A longer TE is likely to make the scan times longer as a longer TR may be needed.
- Try it and see what the radiologists think of it.
- Try fat-sat, that will further cancel signal from background tissue, but may add to the TR.
- MT on pediatric MRAs may trip SAR, and you may need to turn it off.

Flow Compensation

Flow comp should be on all MRAs. Bright blood sequences, MRAs, suffer from something called intra-voxel phase dispersion. This is a signal loss caused by the very fact that blood is moving through a gradient. When tissues pick up phase, they lose signal.

Flow comp is a gradient scheme that minimizes signal loss from moving blood. If a gradient caused a signal loss, a gradient can fix it. See section "Flow Comp" in Chapter 12 for more details.

Another way to get a flow comp effect is to use the shortest TE possible. You do not often see pulsatile artifacts on T1s, except post gadolinium. I am sure you have noticed pulsatile artifacts on T2s and STIRs. Both have long TEs, right?

Teaching Moment: In general, long TR and long TE sequences deserve flow comp in order to minimize the pulsatile artifacts of blood/CSF.

Speaking of flow comp, do you have superior/inferior (S/I) saturation pulses on sagittal T2 and STIR spines? Do you have both flow comp and sats on? If so, then lose (delete) the sats. They are working against each other. Flow comp helps make CSF bright on T2s and STIR, which is a good thing. But sats work to make CSF and other flows dark, like sats for the venous side in an MRA. Sats also add to the patient SAR and may require a longer TR.

Other names for flow compensation are GMR (Gradient Motion Reduction) and GMN (Gradient Motion Nulling).

Phase Contrast MRA

What about the name "phase contrast" (PC)? When you compare two different things to each other, you are said to be "contrasting them." In this instance, we are contrasting phases. Hence the name phase contrast.

PC is common in cardiac imaging to determine flow velocities, a quick "vessel scout" for carotid MRAs, and in CSF flow studies.

PC uses a different method to get its image contrast. Just as TOF angiography relies on vessels being bright and background tissue dark, so too does PC. You will notice that on PC-MRA the background is even darker than it is on TOF.

PC-MRA can be made sensitive to different directions of flow in vessels as well as different flow rates. TOF MRA assumes a constant flow rate, and depending on the direction of flow can actually lose signal in the vessels.

PC has all the same scan factors that TOF angiography has, with one additional factor called "Venc." I shall explain venc later in this section.

Recall that when a magnetic field gradient is applied, all tissues will pick up phase. **Moving tissues pick up even more phase** than stationary tissues. The picking up of additional phase is where we get our contrast in PC-MRA.

When you look at a PC line diagram, it is really a double echo sequence. Here is the skinny: A slice of tissue is excited but an extra pair of gradients is used to induce **phase** in **moving tissue.** An echo is then sampled. **Stationary tissue is not affected by the extra gradient pulses, meaning it picks up no phase.** The process is repeated but with the **extra gradients applied in reversed polarity** or direction, an echo is sampled. Now you have two echoes, each with a different amount of phase. The stationary tissue has a net phase of zero (0) while the moving tissue (blood flow) will have a net phase of something non-zero or plus. In the last step the two echoes are subtracted from each other. The resulting subtraction is: Background tissue is very dark; blood vessels are bright; and you have an MRA data set.

PC is basically a subtraction technique of two TOF MRA echoes. There is a TR, TE, and F/A but an extra scan parameter called "venc," or velocity encoding. The venc is a number, in cm/s, that you enter according to the vessel/flow rate you want to see, meaning is it fast or slow?

- A high venc will visualize fast arterial flow; a low venc is used for slower venous flow; while a very low venc is used in CSF flow studies.
- **Venc numbers:** A high venc is approximately 90+ cm/s for carotids, while a low venc is about 20–30 cm/s. Brain MRV and CSF flow studies typically use a 2–7 venc.
- It is important that you enter the correct venc into the sequence. The venc is the **maximum flow velocity expected** during the acquisition.

The venc you enter adjusts the gradient applications to see up to a certain flow velocity. If the venc is set too low, you will get an artifact called "aliasing." Aliasing happens when the venc is too low because the scanner is looking for a certain flow rate, but the actual rate was higher. The subtraction cannot tell the difference between flow that is faster or slower than the venc and thinks it is stationary tissue. This will be displayed as low signal. Aliasing looks like a dark hole (multiple dark pixels) in a bright vessel, a donut as it were. The sequence will need to be re-run with a better venc, and that takes time.

Some PC sequences can have a long scan time. You can choose which direction to see flow, in the S/I, R/L, or

A/P direction. Each additional direction adds time to the sequence, or you can choose all three at once (an even longer sequence). Scanning in one direction is a much shorter sequence. For example, for a simple flow pattern like in the carotids, pick S/I and it will be a rather short sequence, but a PC in the COW, with its complex flow pattern, needs all three directions. That will take more time. One "knock" against using PC is that if you pick a wrong venc, the sequence needs to be run again with a different venc and exam time goes up.

PC PSDs are shown in Figures 8.13 and 8.14.

> **Teaching Moment:** For the carotid arteries, a quick sagittal or coronal PC is often acquired to serve as a "vessel scout" to help localize the carotid bifurcation. Some technologists use C3/4 as their "go to" spot for the carotid bifurcations.

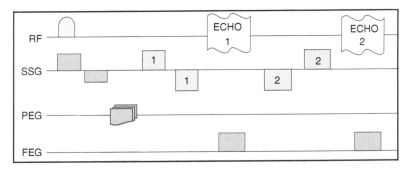

Figure 8.13 PSD of a PC sequence. Note that, in this example, the SSG is applied three times. Gradients labelled 1 produce echo #1, SSG 2 produces echo #2. These two echoes are then subtracted to produce a PC image.

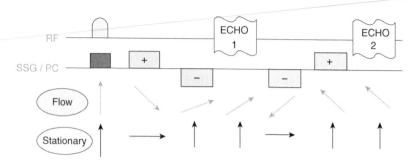

Figure 8.14 A PC PSD. The NMVs for flow and stationary tissue are shown starting at zero at the time of excitation. The first PC gradient causes some amount of "phase" in the tissues which is corrected for by the second PC gradient at the TE (echo 1). For the second TE (echo 2), the gradient scheme is reversed. Note that the **stationary tissue is always at zero** at both the TEs and will be very dark, but **flowing blood is never at zero at the TE.** This means flowing will be bright on the resulting data set.

Sometimes when doing PC it is trial and error unless you are very experienced at it. You will develop a skill set on judging what venc to use. Flow velocity changes from patient to patient due to age, cardiac function, and other underlying medical conditions.

Teaching Moment: PC is not sensitive to the T1 of blood like TOF. If for some reason you miss the timing of a CE-MRA, all hope is not lost. Hopefully you have a 2D or 3D TOF as backup. If not, try a PC. PC does not care about the T1 of blood, which is now shortened by the gadolinium. It gets its contrast from the different amount of phase in the echoes.

Teaching Moment: TOF MRA is a staple in MR. That being said, though, the gold standard for vascular imaging is catheter angiography. The next best is CE-MRA. Why? Both catheter arteriograms and CE-MRA are what is called **"lumenograms,"** meaning that we are directly imaging the **lumen** of the vessel with contrast. TOF MRA is a depiction of flowing spins within the vessels and is fairly accurate for the most part. It does, however, overestimate the size/severity of a narrowing or stenosis whereas contrast angiography does not.

9

k-Space

Chapter at a Glance

"*k*" Is a physics term used to describe frequency. In MR it is used to describe data points in "space," more precisely phase and frequency points. The number of data points is determined by the imaging matrix of a sequence. You might like to relate to *k*-space as a temporary place to put your echoes as they are acquired but before Fourier transform (Figure 9.1). If you have 20 axial slices in the brain then you have 20 *k*-spaces waiting to be filled with echoes from its particular slice. Once the *k*-space(s) is full, Fourier transform takes the data, does the math, and an image is produced, one image for each *k*-space.

MRI Physics: Tech to Tech Explanations, First Edition. Stephen J. Powers.
© 2021 John Wiley & Sons Ltd. Published 2021 by John Wiley & Sons Ltd.

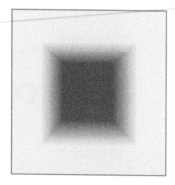

Figure 9.1 A *k*-space. The darker area is the "contrast" portion. Lines in the center zone contribute mostly to image contrast and only a little to image resolution or edge detail. The lighter portion on the outer edge is the "resolution" portion. Lines here contribute mostly to edge detail and a little bit of image contrast.

What Is Fourier Transform?

Fourier transform (FT) is a mathematical algorithm which converts a signal (our echo) into the sum of different amplitudes, phases, frequencies. The data are ultimately processed by the scanner's array processor into the final images.

k-Space Filling

The method by which *k*-space is filled can have a dramatic effect on image contrast. There are multiple ways in which it can be filled. The method changes based on the sequence that is being run. Conventional SE and conventional GRE will use a linear method; FSE/TSE uses a "re-ordered" method. Timed or dynamic sequences use a centric method, and CE-MRA sequences can use one of three methods: Centric, elliptical centric, or "TRICKs/TWIST."

Aside from the linear method, where a line goes in *k*-space will affect the image contrast.

Linear and Re-ordered Filling

Linear filling is shown in Figure 9.2. The *k*-space is filled sequentially line by line, 1, 2, 3, 4, etc. In CSE, **one line of *k*-space** is filled per TR, and **each line has the same TE**. So, it does not really matter where each echo is placed in *k*-space as they all have the same TE (image contrast). Image contrast is not affected by the filling scheme like it can be in FSE.

Re-ordered filling is shown in Figure 9.3. With FSE/TSE multiple TEs (different contrasts) are acquired per TR. Each TE needs to fill a different line of *k*-space. This is where you need to manage the image contrast. The desired image contrast or effective TE (ETE) is placed into the center lines. This requires the amplitudes of the PEG to be altered to place those ETEs in center lines for optimum image contrast while the least desirable TEs will be placed in the outer lines to contribute mostly to resolution or edge detail and the least to image contrast.

Contrast Enhanced MRA

Contrast MRA sequences are T1 weighted GRE sequences. As already stated, there are multiple ways to fill *k*-space. The use of centric and elliptical centric are the common methods in CE-MRA, while dynamic studies typically use centric filling.

Remember that the center lines contribute the most to the image contrast, so how and when we fill those lines, along with timing the arrival of IV contrast, is key for a good CE-MRA/dynamic tissue study.

Centric Filling

Centric filling is shown in Figure 9.4. The central lines are filled first, followed by the outer lines. This is a typical filling scheme for MRAs in the abdomen and pelvis, and dynamic imaging of the liver/renal system/breast. The goal of centric filling is to have the gadolinium arrive at the target vessel/organ with the start of

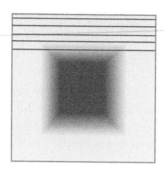

Figure 9.2 Linear filling (CSE or conventional GREs).

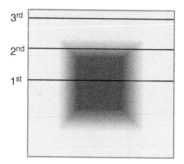

Figure 9.3 Re-ordered filling where, say, line #1 is filled first with the ETE for contrast and line #3 a later TE which contributes resolution (edge detail).

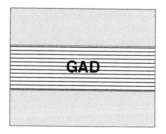

Figure 9.4 Centric filling of k-space, in which the center lines are ideally filled at the same time as gadolinium arrives at the target vessel/organ.

filling the center lines of k-space. There are multiple methods to accomplish this timing. One way is to simply inject and count to "20 Mississippi," which is very unscientific and fraught with inconsistencies such as cardiac output, injection rate, and tech to tech counting speed. There are more reliable methods.

Timing the Arrival of Gadolinium

There are three ways:

1. The old fashioned *"timing bolus"* (Figure 9.5). Inject a 2 ml (cc) bolus of contrast and run a single axial slice just above the target vessel repeatedly for, say, 45–60 s. Each slice takes about 1 s to produce and when the artery you want to image gets bright, that is your scan delay for centric filling.

   The timing bolus method has fallen out of favor because concerns about nephrogenic systemic fibrosis (NSF) and glomerular flow rate (GFR) mandate the smallest dose possible. If you are only injecting 14 ml for the run and giving 2 ml for the timing, that is 14% of your dose for timing. That is a big chunk of the dose.

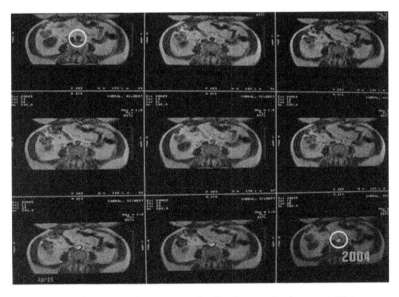

Figure 9.5 A timing bolus run. Each slice is at a 2 s interval. This equates to an 18 s scan delay for the start of data acquisition. Contrast arrival is circled on the bottom right image.

Newer methods to time the arrival of gadolinium are offered by multiple vendors, ranging from fluoroscopic type sequences to a sequence that detects changes in signal intensity when the gadolinium bolus arrives.

2. ***The fluoroscopic type sequence*** (Figure 9.6). This method runs a plane of your choice. The scanner will run the same slice repeatedly as you inject the bolus; watch for the arrival of the gadolinium. When it arrives, you start the sequence. It is like a timing bolus except that you are watching it happen in real time while giving the entire dose of gadolinium. It works very well but careful attention is needed to the progression of gadolinium as it courses through the vasculature. I like to scan these coronally as I can follow visually gadolinium's progression, allowing me to anticipate the start of data acquisition.

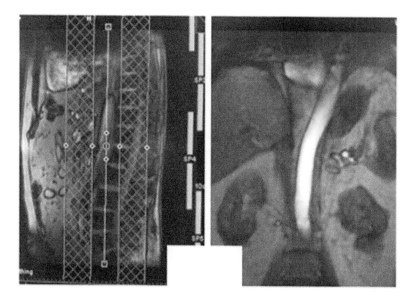

Figure 9.6 A coronal "Fluoro-Trigger" type image in the abdomen. Gadolinium is in the left ventricle and aorta. Some systems save the images to be used as a teaching tool.

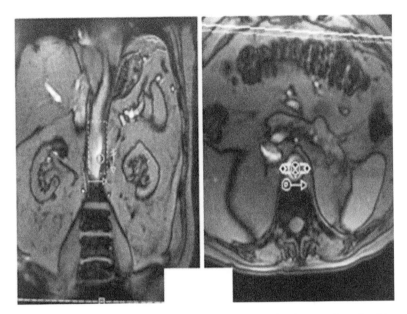

Figure 9.7 The "bolus track/care-bolus" method, where a "tracker" is placed in the target vessel.

3. *The "bolus track/care-bolus"* (Figure 9.7) is where you place a "tracker" in the target vessel. The scanner monitors for a large increase in signal intensity indicating contrast's arrival. **The scanner initiates data acquisition at this point.**

Methods 2 and 3 are "one-time only" timing methods. There is one chance to capture the gadolinium in target vessel.

Elliptical Centric Filling

Elliptical centric filling starts by filling the center lines, rotating its way to the outer lines. This happens because of rotating oscillations of the phase and frequency gradients. The start of the sequence needs to coincide with the arrival of gadolinium. This sequence is commonly used for a carotid MRA (Figures 9.8 and 9.9).

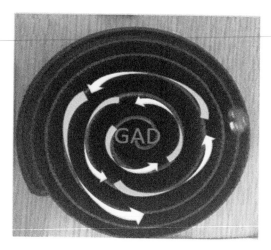

Figure 9.8 Elliptical centric *k*-space filling. Ideally, central lines are filling when gadolinium arrives in the target vessel.

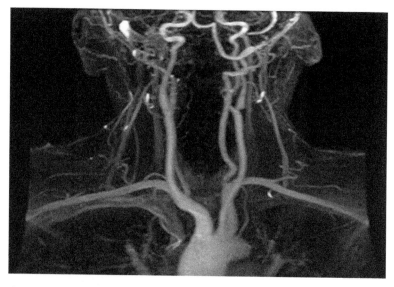

Figure 9.9 Elliptical centric *k*-space filling of the carotids. Inject in the right arm (if possible) as the right subclavian vein does not cross the midline, which could possibly obscure the origins of the great vessels. Vascular disease is not always at or near the carotid bifurcations.

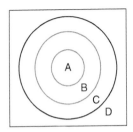

Figure 9.10 The TRICKS/TWIST sequences are even more gradient intense than elliptical centric filling. Think of it as *k*-space being broken into four zones: A, B, C, and D. "A" is the center most with "D" the outermost. As you already know, the center of *k*-space contributes mostly to image contrast while the outer gives the most to resolution. These sequences or filling schemes are "time-resolved" or dynamic acquisitions.

TRICKS/TWIST/4D TRAK

The TRICKS/TWIST sequence is easy to understand. With these sequences, think of *k*-space as broken up into four sections or zones, A, B, C, and D, as shown in Figure 9.10. This sequence has an extra aspect that needs to be explained: Temporal resolution. Temporal relates to or is a way to express **t**ime.

Temporal Resolution and Phases

Temporal resolution is how long it takes to scan the zones. It is usually expressed in seconds. The importance of having a fast or short temporal resolution is that the shorter the temporal resolution is, the less likely it is that you will miss the arrival of the gadolinium.

TRICKS/TWIST sequences scan "phases." A single "phase" consists of scanning the zones in this order; A, B, A, C, A, D. You will likely run 15–30 phases. Temporal resolution is how many seconds it takes to get back to zone "A." The faster you can get back to "A," the better the chance you will have gadolinium in the target vessel and get a good MRA. If the temporal resolution is 4 s, it takes 4 s to scan A, then scan B (4 s), then go back to A for 4 s, then move to C, then back to A, and finally to

D. The math: one phase takes 24 s: $6 \times 4 = 24$. You keep going back to "A," and you should repeat the phase about 10–30 times. Temporal resolution is more important than the time of each phase. A phase time of, say, 40 s or more is too long for an MRA. You will likely get venous contamination. A reasonable time for a phase is 24 s.

Factors Affecting Temporal Resolution

Multiple factors affect temporal resolution. Anything that affects the TR will ultimately affect the temporal resolution:

- Number of locations per slab.
- Fat-sat.
- Phase and frequency matrix.
- TE (keep as short as possible).
- Nex or Acquisition.
- Phase FOV.
- FOV.
- Partial nex of fractional echo.
- Receiver B/W (Hz/pix).

How Do I Know What the Temporal Resolution Should Be?

There is no formula. Just know that the closer to the heart, the faster the blood flow will be, so the shorter the temporal resolution needs to be.

The items listed in the previous section all have an effect on the TR. What I mean by that is, they all make the minimum TR longer, thus increasing the temporal resolution.

General Numbers for Scanning: Carotids: 3–4 s, Arm/hand 5–6 s, Lower legs 6'7 s. Longer temporal resolution means there is more chance to miss the gadolinium in target vessel(s).

There needs to be balance between good temporal resolution, SNR, and spatial resolution. Be sure to evaluate your Pre phase for good coverage, SNR, and artifact. If you have any doubts, adjust and rerun it.

If the temp resolution is short enough, the only reason to miss the gadolinium is if you do not acquire enough phases or forget to connect the injector.

Spatial Resolution

Now let's talk **spatial resolution**. Spatial resolution is basically your pixel size. Spatial resolution does affect temporal resolution. Remember that a high matrix of both phase and frequency costs time whether you are scanning an MRA or the internal auditory canals (IACs). High spatial resolution means a higher temporal resolution.

When scanning these angiography sequences, you do not really need to be concerned with timing the arrival of gadolinium. Run your Pre sequence, check IQ for coverage, SNR, and artifacts. If all those are good, inject and start scanning at the same time.

Some people refer to these angiography sequences as "MRA for Dummies" because it is not hard to get a good angiogram. I hate that saying. I prefer to call it "Run and Gun." Run in the gadolinium (inject), and gun (scan) as fast as you can. With this method, there is no timing sequence. You are hoping gadolinium is in the target vessel when you are scanning zone A/B.

Notes

10

Echo Planar Sequences

Chapter at a Glance

MRI Physics: Tech to Tech Explanations, First Edition. Stephen J. Powers.
© 2021 John Wiley & Sons Ltd. Published 2021 by John Wiley & Sons Ltd.

This chapter will explain the different Echo Planar Imaging (EPI) based sequences. EPI means that a slice's k-space is filled with one 90° RF pulse in one TR period. EPIs have a long string of frequency encoding gradient reversals (Figure 10.1). Each reversal causes an echo which fills a line of k-space. EPI sequences are very gradient intense and very loud.

Besides being loud, they suffer from the same artifacts as a standard GRE, only worse. After all, the echoes produced come from gradient reversals just like a conventional GRE. Metal and off-center FOVs are especially troublesome. There are three different EPI contrasts: SE, inversion recovery (IR), and GRE.

SE-EPI uses 90°–180° RFs pulses for T2 weighting. An IR-EPI uses a series of 180°, –90°, –180° RF pulses for T1 weighting. The GRE-EPI has a 90° RF (but no 180° pulse). GRE-EPI is often used for perfusion studies, taking advantage of the effects of the metallic properties of the gadolinium molecule.

EPIs are very useful as they have a diverse set of applications. This chapter covers the following sequences:

- Diffusion weighted imaging (DWI).
- Diffusion tensor tractography (DTI).
- Susceptibility weighted imaging (SWI) or SWAN.
- Perfusion, or dynamic susceptibility of contrast (DSC).
- Arterial spin labeling (ASL).
- Spectroscopy.

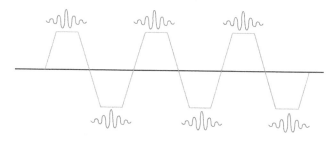

Figure 10.1 An EPI PSD with a string of gradient reversals and resulting echoes.

EPIs are not usually very high resolution because of the very long string of gradient reversals, and are prone to artifacts because they are GRE based even though some of them start off with a SE 90°and 180° RF pulse scheme. Resolution is given up for speed. Even the SE-EPI with one 180° is artifact prone. EPIs can have over 100 gradient reversals, while an FSE can have 20 or more echoes ($\geq$20 180°s). The artifacts commonly seen are chemical shift and distortions (warping) from field inhomogenieties.

Diffusion Weighted Imaging

DWI is a staple in stroke(cerebrovascular accident, CVA) detection and is now commonly used for detecting cancer. A stroke can show diffusion changes as soon as 1 h post ictus versus $\geq$5 h for CT. Our T2s can take up to 10–12 h. DWIs are T2 weighted if you go by the classic long TR and TE, but DWIs have another scan parameter known as a "b" value. b0 will be explained shortly. Actually, DWI gives you a set of T2 images as part of the sequence. It is called the "b0." "Diffusion" weighting is another way of describing image contrast. A T1 image comes from differences in T1 relaxation, a T2 from differences in T2 relaxation. DWI contrast comes from differences in **tissue diffusion.** Tissues with different diffusions have DW contrast.

The word **diffusion** can have multiple meanings to different people, but in MRI think of it as cells **moving** chemicals in and out of themselves to maintain homeostasis (meaning keeping themselves happy and healthy).

> **The Sodium Pump:** When cells have a blood supply (fuel) they can do the work of diffusion via the "sodium pump." When that blood supply is halted, the pump runs out of fuel. When they stop moving materials in and out of themselves, cells start to fill with water and swell. This is called "restricted diffusion." Cells can pop like a balloon and die if the blood supply is not re-established in time.

Movement is key in DWI. By this I mean cellular movement, not gross movement of the patient, which will completely destroy a DWI sequence. You want the cells to be pumping (diffusing) chemicals and fluids in and or out.

How DWI Works

Earlier I stated that tissues moving through or in the presence of a magnetic field gradient will pick up phase (see "Phase Contrast MRA" in Chapter 8). When tissues pick up phase, they actually lose the ability to generate a lot of signal. Here is the key concept in DWI: **Diffusing tissue (cellular movement) picks up phase and will be darker than the non-moving tissue (the CVA), which will not pick up any phase and will be bright**. On DWI weighted images you are looking for a bright area in the brain that represents a lack of cellular diffusion (restricted movement). Normal tissue is darker. If treated quickly enough, a CVA's effects can at least be minimized.

A basic DWI sequence will produce four data sets:

- A T2 or b_0 which is a low resolution T2 weighted image. You can think of this as a "control" in the MR experiment. The b_0 (T2) comes from running the sequence without any diffusion gradients.
- The other three data sets, which you do not usually see, have "diffusion gradients" applied in the three cardinal directions: Slice, phase, and frequency. Diffusion happening in each of the three directions will be slightly darker than tissue that is not diffusing. When one tissue is bright (the stroke), next to another (normal) which is dark, this equals **contrast, actually diffusion contrast or DWI.**

So, what is all this talk about diffusion? How is an image "diffused"? It is done with a pair of gradients applied **one just before the 180° and one just after, but before the TE.** The echo will contain diffusion contrast. Figure 10.2 shows what it looks like in a line diagram.

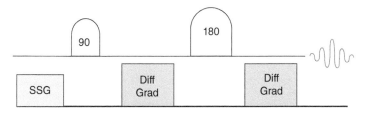

Figure 10.2 A stripped-down PSD of a DWI sequence showing DW gradients, here applied in the SSG direction. Here diffusion in the **slice** direction will be darker than others.

What Is the "b-Value"?

The "b-value" is a number used to describe the amount of diffusion caused by the gradients. It is used to describe how sensitive a sequence is to detecting a stroke. A high b-value means a lot of diffusion with increased sensitivity to restricted diffusion (stroke). A low b-value number is a lesser amount of diffusion and a lower sensitivity to restricted diffusion. **Restricted diffusion** means cells are not moving fluids in and out normally. The standard definition of b-value is: A value representing the amplitude (strength) and or duration (time) of the applied diffusion gradients (Figure 10.3). In layman's terms: **long or strong is a high b-value; short or weak is a low b-value.**

DWI FYIs

- Diffusion is a thermodynamic and non-equilibrium driven process that moves waste, nutrients, and dissolved gases into and out of a cell. High concentrations move to lower concentrations, like heat in your home.
- Diffusion is driven by a tissue's perfusion (blood supply). Perfusion stops, diffusion stops.
- When diffusion stops, a tissue's signal increases because the sodium pump stopped working.

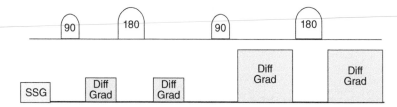

Figure 10.3 Gradients for a low b-value on the left and high b-value on the right. Remember height = amplitude or strength while length or duration of application is time running left to right. An echo acquired after the right diffusion gradients would be more sensitive to stroke compared to an echo after the left gradients.

Teaching Moment: The higher the b-value, the more phase dispersion happens but the lower the overall SNR. A higher b-value needs more Nex or averages to buy back that SNR.

Teaching Moment: One b-value does not fit all. A b-value of 1000 is typical in the brain. Some facilities use 1200–1500 in the brain to increase sensitivity. In the liver/pancreas, a b-value of 700 or 800 is common. In the prostate, a 1400 b-value is standard with lots of nex as the FOVs and slice thicknesses are pretty small so signal is at a premium.

Teaching Moment: TR has little to do with image contrast in DWI, so use the minimum. DW contrast comes from the b-value plus TE. Keep the TE as short as possible to help with SNR.

So why are there different b-values? The answer is: Different tissue structure. The brain has a "sponge" like consistency and diffuses easily. Liver/pancreas are more "jelly" like and diffuse more easily than the brain. The prostate is denser so cellular diffusion is not so easy. The b-values given previously are common numbers but your radiologists will have their own preferences for b-values. Check with them before making protocol changes.

DWI: Summary: Tissues that are not perfused (stroking) have no cellular diffusion going on and the tissues do not de-phase from the applied DW gradients. They will be bright when compared to the perfused/diffusing tissue which is dark.

The bright area in Figure 10.4 is an acute CVA, b-1000. It is bright as the tissue is not being perfused so cellular diffusion has stopped. Normal tissue is darker by comparison, and has a lower signal due to phase acquired from the DW gradients. If it is not moving, it will not pick up phase and will be bright,

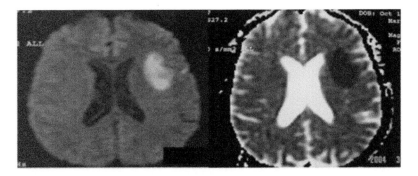

Figure 10.4 Acute CVA in the left parietal lobe; b-value 1000. Apparent diffusion coefficient (ADC) map (same slice) on the right. Remember: Bright on b_0 and dark on ADC = stroke.

that is, diffusion weighted. While not SAR intense, DWIs are very gradient intense so peripheral nerve stimulation (PNS) is a possibility. DWIs are also very loud because of rapid gradient switching. Being GRE based, everything that will affect a regular GRE will also affect a DWI but more so. Metal from dentures or from corrective braces is a killer.

A real-life demonstration of diffusion is shown in Figure 10.5, axial images acquired during a prostate exam. An incidental finding of a bladder diverticulum was made. What is demonstrated is a jet of urine between the actual bladder and the diverticulum. It is seen on all three weightings: T2, B_0, and an 800 b-value. Note that the moving urine picks up phase and loses signal as it moves. Signal loss actually increases from the T2 to the b_0 and is maximum in the b-800. Each is progressively more sensitive to the de-phasing from the urine flow. This is a good example of what happens in the brain during a CVA. Perfused tissues with a working sodium pump (diffusion) are slightly darker when compared to tissues with less diffusion, which are bright. In this bladder, stagnant urine is bright, meaning **it did not acquire phase** from the DW gradients, while the jet of moving urine picks up phase, hence signal loss.

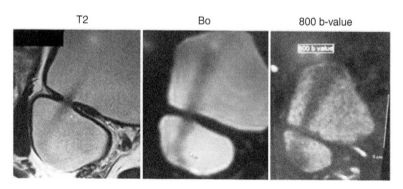

Figure 10.5 A bladder diverticulum found during a prostate study. Note signal loss on each side from flowing urine, especially on the b-800. This is a good example of the signal loss (de-phasing) resulting from movement.

What Is an Apparent Diffusion Coefficient (ADC) Map?

Another set of images produced in a DWI sequence is the "apparent diffusion coefficient" map (Figure 10.6). When you put a tea bag in water, the tea will spread out or diffuse into the water until equilibrium is reached. Water is a homogeneous medium compared to the human body. The tea will "diffuse" or blend into the water at a certain **rate** that varies with the temperature, flow, or viscosity of the medium. That rate is called the diffusion coefficient. The human body is anything but uniform, so cellular diffusion is far from easy or straightforward. ADC maps are basically a visual representation of the "estimated" or **apparent** diffusion of the tissues. There is no number with which to quantify it. Being a visual representation, a dark area means that very little to no diffusion happened. It should correspond very nicely to the bright area on the b-1000 images. In other words, is the bright area on the b-1000 the same shape, size, and location as the dark area on the ADC?

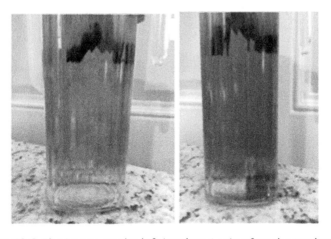

Figure 10.6 The image on the left is taken 1 min after the tea bags were placed in water, that on the right about 5 min later. Note that the tea has diffused almost fully.

It is easy to remember which is which, and on which image:

bright on the **b**-1000, and **D**ark on the A**D**C map = stroke.

An ADC map is calculated by putting signal intensities of the pixels through the Stejskal–Tanner equation. For that equation to work, **you need at least two b-values for the math to give you the ADC map.** It is likely that your DWI sequences are saved in protocol with two b-values (say b-0 and b-1000) so you will not even have to think of needing two b-values.

Teaching Moment: You can do a DWI sequence with just a single b-value. Simply tell the scanner to do one b-value and it will do it; just do not go looking for, or try to manually create an ADC map.

How and Why Is an ADC Map Used/Needed?

The ADC map acts as a confirmation (a tie breaker) for the radiologists to call a bright area a stroke. A bright area on the b-1000 is usually a CVA. If an area in question is dark on the ADC map and bright on the DWI, it is a CVA. That is an easy call.

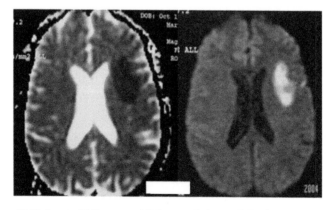

Figure 10.7 Acute CVA on an ADC map, left, and the b-1000 DWI image right. Same slice, same patient.

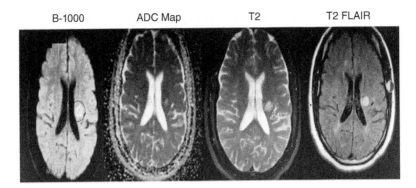

B-1000   ADC Map   T2   T2 FLAIR

Figure 10.8 These images are same slice, same patient. There is a round lesion (circled). It is fairly bright on b-1000. Is this due to restricted diffusion? The lesion is also bright on the ADC map so it is not acting like a stroke. Tissue with decreased or restricted diffusion should be dark on an ADC, right? The T2-weighted image confirms that the brightness on the ADC is the "T2 shine through" effect. It is also bright on the T2 FLAIR and is behaving like an MS plaque. Multiple weightings are needed to determine this pathology. (It is a previously documented MS plaque.)

What if an area is bright on both? Fluid is bright on an ADC map. Look at the ventricles in Figure 10.7. A chronic stroke will be full of CSF and do the "fluid thing" on multiple different weightings, including the ADC map.

Brightness on both images **could** be something called **"T2 shine through,"** which happens when a tissue (e.g. CSF) has a **very long T2 time**. It looks as if it has restricted diffusion on DWI, even though it does not. T2 shine through it is not a CVA. It is described in more detail in the next section.

T2 Shine Through

Let's look at Figure 10.8. The circled ROI on the b-1000 could be a CVA. On the ADC and T2 images it is doing the "fluid thing." If that is really true, why is fluid **bright** on the T2 FLAIR? FLAIR (fluid attenuated inversion recovery) is supposed to have dark fluid, as in the ventricles? What gives?

The fluid (edema) in the MS plaque has a different T1 relaxation time compared to the T1 of CSF. It is fluid but it is not the same fluid as in the ventricles. CSF is mostly water so the TI used to suppress CSF will not work on the plaque edema. That TI is too long. **Recall,** a long TI suppresses long T1 tissue, and a short TI suppresses short T1 tissue. Examples of short T1 relaxing tissues are **fat, gadolinium, and protein (edema is a proteinaceous fluid),** and long T1 tissues are **CSF and urine.**

The eADC Map: Exponential ADC

An exponential ADC map is another way to remove any T2 contrast from the images. In reality, it is the b_0 image **divided by the DW image. It is a calculated image that removes T2 shine through effects on DWIs.** Call it another tie breaker, if you like, to answer the clinical question of T2 shine through or not (Figure 10.9). A radiologist may still have doubts that an ROI is T2 shine through on the T2, ADC, and B_0 images. Compared to the ADC map, it is a reversed contrast image where **all "T2 contrast" is removed mathematically** by the above-mentioned post processing. eADC maps remove T2 shine through. **Remember,** an image does not have to be pretty to answer the clinical question. If the clinical question is answered, then it is beautiful.

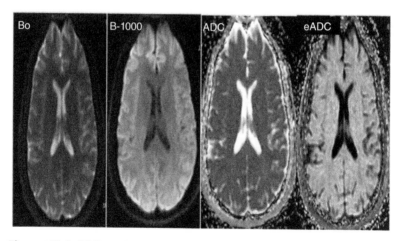

Figure 10.9 All four DWI images next to each other. Images are the same slice and same patient.

Diffusion Tensor Imaging or White Matter Tractography

Conventional DWI in the brain typically diffuses (applies DW gradients) in three to six directions: R/L, A/P, S/I. Diffusion tensor imaging (DTI) is DWI on steroids. DTI is DWI with 6 to more than 27 DW gradient direction applications. More directions mean a longer scan time.

DTI lets you image the different WM tracts by their direction of diffusion. These images come from the fact that WM tracts run in and through the brain like bundles of wires. Diffusion (flow) does not cross the WM cell membranes well, but it does diffuse (flow) along or within WM tracts rather well (like blood flow in a vessel). Figure 10.10 shows examples of WM tracts in color.

Think of DTI as being like a TOF MRA for WM tracts. While scanning, some DW directions will be **parallel** to various WM tracts and the diffusion running along those tracts will lose signal and not be seen well (in-plane saturation). The opposite is also true. Some directions of DW will be at **a right angle** (90°) to a WM tract, and **it will appear bright** (the TOF effect). The DTI sequence runs with many, many directions, and you are bound to be at right angles to any of them at one time or another. This is why the more directions you run in a DTI sequence the better (more) you see the tracts. DTI usually has 20–27 directions, but if you go to 50 directions, for example, it shows you more fibers.

Figure 10.10A is a Christmas ornament but it equates to or depicts the many directions in a DTI sequence.

DTI or white matter tractography can be useful in presurgical planning to show WM tract infiltration or deflection from a tumor. In trauma situations, color maps can help define the severity of diffuse traumatic brain injury. Color maps show the direction of diffusion: Red is R/L, blue is S/I, and green is A/P. 3D color maps can be rotated for more projections.

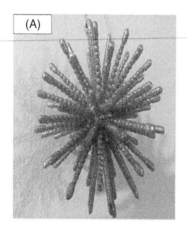

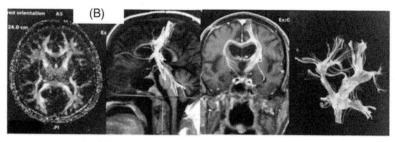

Figure 10.10 A. The many directions in a DTI sequence. Each "arm" in the ornament is a diffusion direction. B. Diffusion tensor images. Left. A directional map: Red means diffusion is R/L; green is A/P; and blue is S/I. Middle. The WM tracts are superimposed on the accompanying patient images. Right. Image of the WM tracts alone without background anatomy.

Susceptibility Weighted Imaging

GRE based sequences are sensitive to differences in magnetic "susceptibility" between tissues. Some sequences take it to a higher level. Different vendors, of course, have different names for these EPI based sequences: Siemens = SWI; GE = SWAN;

Philips: Venous BOLD. EPI (echoplanar imaging) means that they are extra sensitive to susceptibility because the echoes come from gradient reversals, not 180°'s. Basically, they are DWIs without the diffusion gradients. If you think about it, the conventional GRE commonly run during a brain exam is really susceptibility weighted. It is just not referred to as such. Susceptibility weighted images go by different names and can be to referred as iron axials, T2*s, T2 star, susceptibility axials, trauma axials, etc. Everybody seems to have a different name for them but they all mean the same thing: They are sensitive to local magnetic susceptibilities.

True susceptibility weighted sequences are EPI sequences and are even more sensitive to the effects of hemorrhage. These SWI sequences are higher in resolution than the standard GRE sequence as they are trying to see petechial (small) hemorrhages (Figures 10.11 and 10.12).

As already stated, SWI images are used to identify hemorrhage. These are fairly high resolution compared to other EPIs because they are used to identify post-traumatic petechial hemorrhages. Look at the vessels on the images in Figure 10.13. Conventional GRE does not really show any vasculature, whereas the SWIs do.

Small bleeds from trauma/concussion will show as small dark areas of **susceptibility** very close to the vessels. As you know, brain tissue does not have a true blood supply because of the blood–brain barrier (BBB).

Typical scan parameters for a SWI is: 3D with 2–3 mm thick partitions, high matrix: 256×256, 3–4 Nex/ACQ for SNR, scan time often 3–4 min. This is quite long for an EPI sequence, but it is a high-resolution sequence and that takes time. A 3D sequence offers a higher SNR, the ability to reformat, and thinner slices. SWI reformats are minimum intensity projection or minimum IP to make the vessels dark. MRA uses maximum IP, or MIP to make vessels bright.

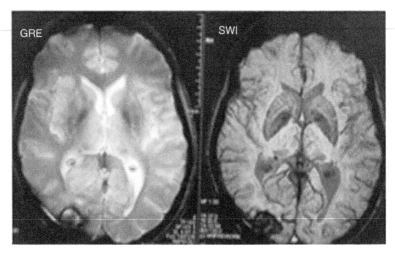

Figure 10.11 You are looking for blood to cause a small local field inhomogeneity/susceptibility artifact. Same image GRE and SWI on top. Note the right occipital lobe.

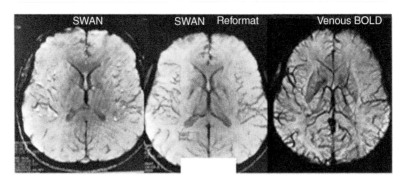

Figure 10.12 Multiple images of a sequence known as SWI, SWAN, and Venous BOLD. All are used to detect small hemorrhages in the brain from trauma. Compare with the standard GRE axial in Figure 10.11.

Brain Perfusion

The word perfusion means different things to different people. Another word or description for an MR perfusion study is "dynamic susceptibility of contrast" or (DSC). It can also be described as first-pass DSC. In MR, DSC shows how much of

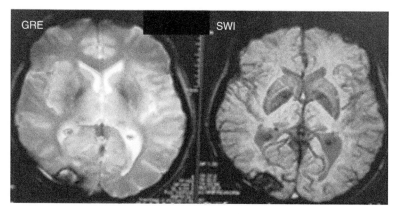

Figure 10.13 A standard GRE next to a high resolution SWI.

the brain is being affected by a lack of blood flow. The main premise of doing a perfusion study is to visualize the area that has been affected by a stroke but, more importantly, to detect an area that is on the verge of also becoming or extending a CVA and can be saved.

When a CVA is occurring, there are two parts or zones to the actual stroke: The umbra and the penumbra. The **umbra** is that part that **is dying or dead**. The **penumbra** is an area that is on the edge of dying and **can be saved** through medical treatment.

Here is the skinny on DSC. It is a 3D sequence that is run many times (say ≥30) in rapid succession. Each run or phase is perhaps 7–10 s. Several phases are run before injecting the contrast. When the gadolinium arrives, the perfused tissue will drop in signal intensity. Gadolinium, being a metal, will cause a small amount of susceptibility in the tissue, resulting in a small amount of signal loss. The non-perfused tissue that does not receive any gadolinium will not change in signal. As in a DWI, perfused tissue drops in signal, non-perfused tissue is bright.

A word about the gadolinium injection: 99.9% of the time, you are using the T1 relaxivity of gadolinium, but in DSC you are using the T2 relaxivity of gadolinium.

There are various post processing techniques, as well as several color maps depicting different timings and tissue qualities. These maps and values are: **mean transit time (MTT), time to peak (TTP), relative cerebral blood flow (rCBF), and relative cerebral blood volume (rCBV).** The word "relative" is used as it is difficult to quantify these qualities with great accuracy. **MTT** is the time it takes for the gadolinium bolus to reach (transit) the brain. **TTP** is the time for the maximum amount of signal loss. Those two you can get easily from the graph in Figure 10.14.

The next two are color maps with red representing a lot of gadolinium and blue less. **rCBF is the "relative"** amount of cerebral blood flow. This is usually the most important of all the four maps. Finally, the **rCBV** represents the relative cerebral blood volume. rCBV is usually used in tumor characterization.

Figure 10.15 shows a known stroke (large arrow). On this perfusion (DSC) image, a round ROI is placed #1 with the accompanying signal intensity graph also labeled #1 on the right. The signal intensity is very low as expected and the graph does

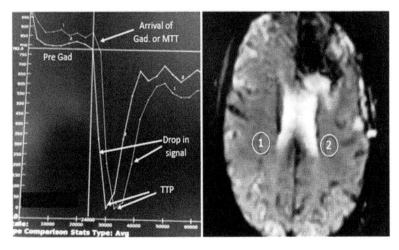

Figure 10.14 Brain perfusion graphs (not for diagnostic purposes).

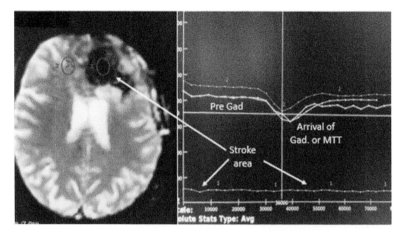

Figure 10.15 The graph shows the signal intensity of ROI #2 (right frontal) before arrival of the IV contrast. At the arrival of the contrast, there is a drop in signal due to the susceptibility changes caused by the arrival of the gadolinium. The very bottom of the graph is listed left to right in milliseconds to get the MTT and TTP values. Also shown is the signal intensity of two ROIs before and during arrival of the gadolinium. ROI right frontal #2 shows a normal curve while curve #1 left frontal is all but flat, depicting very little to no flow due to no blood supply. Note the line at the bottom of the graph. Yes, this is an old CVA and, yes, the ROI was placed there knowing no flow would be detected. This was done for effect so that you get the "gad/no gad" effect from perfusion.

not change, demonstrating no contrast perfused into the ROI. The contralateral side (ROI #2) does demonstrate a base-line amount of signal prior to arrival, an expected decrease in signal on arrival of the gadolinium. The drop in signal is due to the metallic properties of the IV gadolinium. The T2 time of the tissue is actually shortened and the SNR of the perfused tissue will drop. These two vastly different perfused sites were chosen for teaching purposes.

Figure 10.16 shows the four different perfusion maps that detail different types of brain perfusion.

Color maps may not visualize well in greyscale.

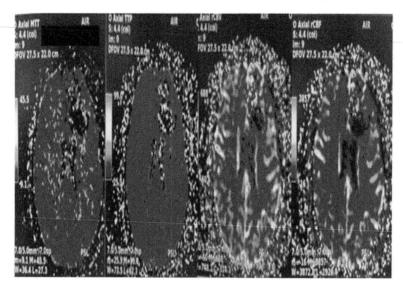

Figure 10.16 Cerebral perfusion maps. Mean transit time (MTT) and time to peak (TPP) are on the left, relative cerebral blood flow (rCBF) and relative cerebral blood volume (rCBV) are on the right. The CVA is easily seen. On the rCBV and rCBF high concentrations of gadolinium are depicted in yellows and reds. Blue is the perfused tissue, black = no perfusion. rCBF maps are used to show CVA and penumbra, while the rCBV is used to show the CVA. As an FYI, GM normally has two to three times as much perfusion as WM.

Arterial Spin Labeling

Arterial spin labeling (ASL) is a **non-contrast** method to show brain perfusion. The ASL's sequence is PD weighted: Long TR, short TE.

ASL works by applying an RF pulse **(the label)** to **arterial** blood **(the spins)** which will then enter the brain (Figure 10.17). You can think of "the label" much like a sat pulse in TOF MRA. These labeled spins can be thought of as "pre-excited" as they travel into the brain. After a predetermined delay time or **Post Labeling Delay (PLD)**, the brain

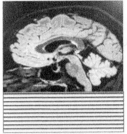 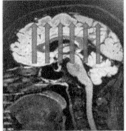 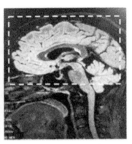

The arterial blood is labeled — During the PLD, labeled spins move into the brain — volume is imaged

Figure 10.17 The different phases or parts of an ASL sequence.

is then imaged. The labeled spins get an additional RF pulse while in the volume and become slightly saturated. Perfused brain will be slightly darker than non-perfused brain. It is a similar idea to the gadolinium perfusion concept except that you do not use any gadolinium. **Do not scan an ASL post gadolinium. ASL is very dependent** on the T1 relaxation of blood.

- The labeling happens inferior to the imaging volume. The PLD allows time for the "labeled" spins to travel into or perfuse the brain.
- ASL acquires two data sets, a non-labeled set and a labeled set. Basically, these are a pre and a post, which are then **subtracted** and the difference between them is shown as a rCBF map.
- Think of the non-labeled images as the "control" in the MR experiment; the labeled image is the variable.
- The weighting in ASL is proton density.
- Tortuous vessels can cause an almost complete loss of signal distal to the tortuosity. Look at the carotid and circle of Willis MRAs.

Rules for ASL: ASL must be done pre contrast. Gadolinium shortens the T1 of blood.

- The patient's head needs to be very straight in all three planes. If it is not, you could get a false positive or negative rCBF. An obliquity changes the distance blood has to travel and ultimately the PLD from side to side.
- Cardiac output affects what PLD you should use: Geriatric vs. pediatric vs. routine patients.
- 1000–1500 ms is a common PLD for pediatric patients; under 1 year a PLD of 500–1000 ms is not uncommon. This may be different in a child with sickle cell or heart disease, in whom the flow is slower and the PLD should be lengthened. At 3–12 years of age a 1250 ms PLD works well.
- In geriatric/heart disease patients with slower flow, a PLD of 2500–3000 ms is average.
- Overall SNR decreases the longer the PLDs.

ASL images are shown in Figure 10.18.

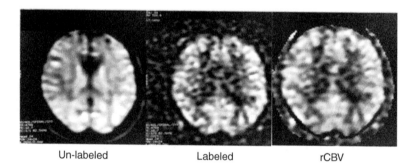

Un-labeled   Labeled   rCBV

Figure 10.18 ASL image: Un-labeled on left, labeled in middle, and rCBV far right. This case was a normal volunteer. No stroke is displayed.

Spectroscopy

Spectroscopy has occasionally been called a biopsy without a needle. **Why?** Because it enables you to get information about a tissue in a non-invasive manner, without needles. Spectroscopy can give you information about disease processes based on the different chemical concentrations within an area or voxel that you placed. **How?** Different disease processes will cause chemical levels to either rise or fall away from normal levels. The different chemicals are called metabolites.

What you are actually doing is scanning an area or voxel in order to get a visible spectrum or set of peaks that tells the radiologist what is going on inside that voxel. The signal from these metabolites is rather small so the area is scanned many times.

Think about this, when you do a manual tuning for fat-sat. Those peaks you see are actually a spectroscopy or spectrum of fat/water frequencies (see Figure 10.19 on the left).

In the brain, where most spectroscopies are performed, the metabolites can be seen in between the fat and water peaks.

Fat and water are different chemicals separated from each other by their specific PFs. The metabolites also have their own PFs that place them between the fat and water peaks (Figure 10.19, right). The arrow points to where the metabolites are between fat and water.

Different disease processes have a "signature" of their own. For example, in tumors, the creatine and choline peaks are

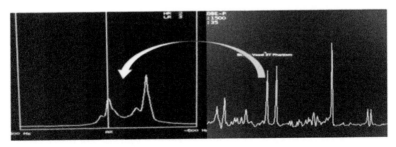

Figure 10.19 A fat-sat tuning spectrum on the left, and an actual spectroscopy showing the various metabolite peaks.

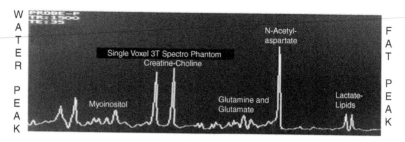

Figure 10.20 Spectroscopy showing peaks of the five most common metabolites.

raised, and the N-acetyl-aspartate (NAA) peak will drop. That is a bad finding. In anoxic brains, lactate and lipids will rise. That is very bad as it is a marker of brain death. The radiologists use these different markers or signatures for diagnostic purposes.

Figure 10.20 shows the five most common and easily identified metabolites. Below is a list and brief descriptions.

- **Lactate–Lipids (LL):** Often called the death peaks. These peaks elevate in states of cell death, tissue necrosis, and anoxic events such as near drowning. At 1.3 ppm.
- **N-Acetyl-aspartate (NAA):** A marker of cell integrity/health and will depress when neurons are being destroyed. At 2.0 ppm, but can drop in cases of MS.
- **Glutamine–Glutamate (GG):** Not usually seen but related to liver function. At 2.1–2.5 ppm.
- **Creatine–Choline (CC):** Referred to as the twin peaks. Usually elevate in the presence of malignancy. At 3.0 and 3.2 ppm.
- **Myoinositol (ml):** A sugar alcohol that elevates in the case of myelin breakdown from Alzheimer's disease and malignancies. Peak is at 3.6 ppm.
- Peaks to the left of myoinositol are unreliable markers, as they are too close to water at 4.0 ppm.

Spectroscopy: Some FYIs

- There are single- and multi-voxel spectroscopy sequences. Single is quicker than multi. It is more reliable and easier to reproduce. Multi is really not much more than a group of singles all run at the same time. Speaking of single voxels, you will need to do two voxels, one in the pathology and the other on the contralateral side for comparison. Do the pathology side first; if the patient refuses to continue, it makes no sense to have just the normal side.
- Spectroscopy is, as I like to say, "crying to fail." When placing your voxel, stay away from bone, blood, surgical clips in the skull, areas of radiation necrosis, and CSF. All of these can cause the spectroscopy to fail or be non-diagnostic. Motion is also a spectroscopy killer. If the patient is confused, has Parkinson's, or for other reasons cannot hold still, forget about it.
- **Spectroscopies can be run post gadolinium** and often are. Sometimes seeing the lesion is difficult without gadolinium. So, for the best chance of a good spectroscopy, perform it post gadolinium.
- Two technical aspects involved in spectroscopy are major concerns: **Water suppression and line width. Water suppression** is just that: An RF pulse is used to null signal from water. With the metabolites being between fat and water, suppression of H_2O is essential. H_2O gives a lot of signal. One of the pre-scan factors in the quality of a spectroscopy is how well or how much water suppression you achieved. The higher the percentage the better. A good suppression is 95% or higher. Below that, the water side of the spectroscopy is high and it works its way down.
- The spectroscopy should have a fairly level baseline from right to left (Figure 10.21, dotted line). If it is tilted then you likely have water contamination. A rather poor spectroscopy shows abnormal baseline from water contamination.

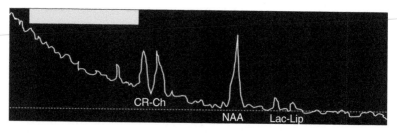

Figure 10.21 Spectroscopy: Water contamination.

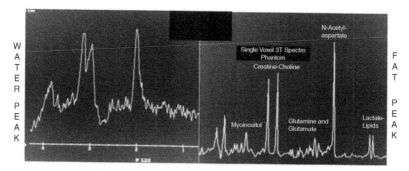

Figure 10.22 On the right is a good spectroscopy, on the left a poor spectroscopy. It is poor because of the "wide" peaks and an elevated baseline.

- The other technical aspect to be concerned with is the **"line width."** This is the distance or "width" from one side of a peak to the other. The smaller the line width (narrow peaks) the better is the spectroscopy. A wide line width lets peaks merge into each other (Figure 10.22). This of concern, especially for the creatine–choline peaks as they are close to each other.

- A neurosurgeon named C. Hunter Shelden used to hold his pocket comb up to a spectroscopy to connect the NAA and creatine–choline peaks (Figure 10.23). If that line from the peak of NAA to the creatine–choline peaks is at approximately 45° then the spectroscopy is mostly normal (Hunter's angle).

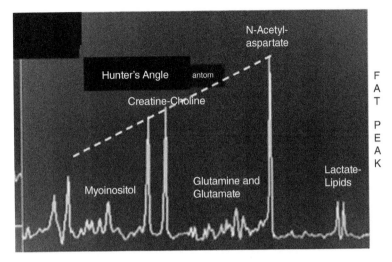

Figure 10.23 "Hunter's angle" in brain spectroscopy.

It is of course not a technologist's job to diagnose anything, but, when doing a brain spectroscopy, it is nice to know what the terms refer to and also what they mean.

Notes

11

Geometric Parameters
Trade-offs and Effects on Image Quality

Chapter at a Glance

MRI Physics: Tech to Tech Explanations, First Edition. Stephen J. Powers.
© 2021 John Wiley & Sons Ltd. Published 2021 by John Wiley & Sons Ltd.

Fractional Echo
Bandwidth
   Receiver Bandwidth
   Transmitter Bandwidth
Rectangular (Rec.) FOV
No Phase Wrap/Phase Oversampling/Fold-over
   Suppression
Concatenations or Acquisitions
Sequential Order Acquisition

Just as image contrast has a "triangle," so too does the image quality (IQ) aspect of MRI (Figure 11.1). Remember from Chapter 3 that **contrast** is the most important aspect of IQ, SNR second, and resolution a close third. **Resolution (spatial resolution) is the number of pixels in the FOV and slice thickness.** This section will cover factors **other** than how TR and TE affect IQ.

Field of View (FOV) Is Your Film Size

FOV is how big your slices are. The FOV runs parallel to the slice select direction and is related not to thickness but to extent in the other two dimensions, which are phase and frequency.

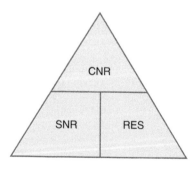

Figure 11.1 The image quality triangle, where contrast to noise (CNR) is the primary consideration with signal to noise (SNR) and resolution being close second and third.

FOV affects multiple aspects of the image: Coverage, SNR, and resolution. **It is a huge contributor to, or killer of SNR.** It can also contribute to the artifact called wrap, aliasing, or fold-over depending on manufacturer.

You need to match your FOV to the body part. Small body parts need a small FOV. FOV terminology or scale varies according to manufacturer terms and is stated in size as either mm or cm (20 cm = 200 mm). It affects multiple aspects of the IQ triangle.

FOV Can Affect Image Contrast

Where does the FOV come from? The FOV comes from the FEG during echo readout. A large FOV means the FEG is applied at a shallower pitch compared to a small FOV, which needs a steeper pitch (Figure 11.2). Also know that a small FOV means the FEG will have to harder and that hard work comes at a price, which is time. Using a small FOV (a steeper pitch) means the FEG needs extra time to come up to strength. A longer TE may result. Have you ever gotten a pop-up saying the minimum TE has been increased by 2 ms? Or maybe a longer TR is needed? That is coming from a small FOV.

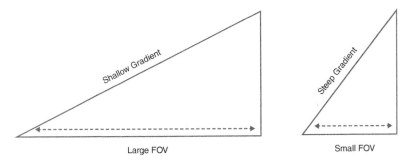

Figure 11.2 The FOV comes from the amplitude or "steepness" of the FEG. A steep or strong gradient means a small FOV whereas a weaker amplitude FEG yields a larger FOV.

Teaching Moment: Does it take you longer to walk up a steep hill or a shallow hill? The steeper one, right? It takes longer for gradients to come up to the "steep" strength. This is called "rise time." TR or TE may need to be lengthened when a small FOV is needed. See Chapter 13 for more information.

So, what difference does a couple of ms make? If you are in T2 land and add 3 ms to a 102 TE there will be little change to contrast, but in T1 land going from 10 ms to 13 ms is a 30% increase and that is a significant jump in TE. Image contrast will change, and fluid will get a bit brighter.

FOV and SNR

Let's say you halve the FOV and go from a 400 to 200 mm. The SNR will drop to one quarter of its original value (from 100% to 25%). That is huge. Wait, I only halved the FOV, why didn't it drop to 50%? The why is: When you halve the FOV, you are decreasing in **two** directions: $\frac{1}{2} \times \frac{1}{2} = \frac{1}{4}$. The opposite also is true. Doubling the FOV increases the SNR fourfold ($2 \times 2 = 4$). Be careful when dropping the FOV: Watch the SNR and also watch the phase direction for wrap. TR and TE may also be affected.

FOV: Pixel Size and SNR

Pixel size is the FOV divided by the scan matrix. A 256 mm FOV with a 256^2 matrix yields a 1×1 mm pixel size: $256 \div 256 = 1$. Again, if you halve the FOV to 128 mm, SNR drops like a stone because the pixel size decreases to 0.5×0.5 mm (halved in two directions). This gives great resolution to be sure, but it does you no good if there is no signal with which to see it. Buying back the SNR means either adding nex (increased scan time) or halving the matrix to 128^2. Resolution returns to 1×1 and SNR returns to close to its original value. **Matrix numbers do not matter, it is pixel size.** Smaller pixels increase resolution but decrease SNR as there are fewer protons per pixel. You need to get pixels in the pathology but balance SNR and resolution.

FOV: Voxel Size and SNR

A voxel is a pixel with a thickness, slice thickness to be exact. "Voxel size" is often mentioned for 3D sequences. **However, 2D sequences also have voxels.** A pixel has two dimensions, height and width; voxels have depth, or a slice thickness.

Often 3D sequences are reformatted into another orthogonal plane. For best reformatting or MIPping an MRA, scanning with isotropic voxels is preferred. **Isotropic** means having the same dimensions in all three directions. A voxel that is $1 \times 1 \times 1$ is isotropic, whereas one that is $1 \times 1 \times 2$ is not, it is **anisotropic**. Most scanners now calculate and display voxel size for you.

- For 3D sequences you want to strive for isotropic voxels. That is easy as slice thickness can easily be 1 mm or less.
- In 2D sequences you seldom if ever have isotropic voxels. That is just not practical SNR wise. All factors being the same, a 3D sequence has a higher SNR than a 2D.

Shortly, I shall talk about and encourage you to scan with square pixels. I shall also explain and encourage the use of a "balanced echo train."

Nex, ACQ, NSA, and SNR

Nex, ACQ, and NSA are vendor acronyms for how many times the k-space will be filled. In a 256^2 matrix with 1 nex you are telling the scanner to fill the k-space once, 2 nex, fill it twice. Going from 1 to 2 nex, the scan time will double but SNR only goes up to a factor of 1.4. It is not a 1:1 ratio. Some sequences will allow a ½ or ¾ nex. These are CE-MRAs where a short scan time is a major concern.

- SNR increases by the square root ($\sqrt{}$) of the number of averages.
- The $\sqrt{}$ of 1 = 1, $\sqrt{}$ of 2 = 1.4, $\sqrt{}$ of 3 = 1.7, and finally the $\sqrt{}$ of 4 = 2. So, it takes four times the scan time to double the SNR. This is not an efficient way to get more signal.

A nex, NSA, etc. is the number of times the scanner will fill each line of k-space. So why, when I double my nex, does the SNR not double? Earlier in the book, I said that signal is something that we make happen. Consider it a "constant" as it were. Every time we make an echo, it is a finite and constant amount of signal for that particular sequence. Noise on the other hand, while always present in all electronic equipment, **constantly varies in amount or intensity**. So, during the first nex, noise may be lower than during the second nex. They average out to the square root ($\sqrt{}$) of the number of nex (Figures 11.3 and 11.4).

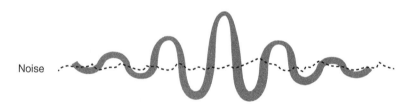

Figure 11.3 Noise (the dotted line) has a lower amplitude than the signal for good SNR.

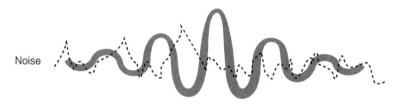

Figure 11.4 For the second nex, the amplitude of the noise is higher so SNR is lower. Also note that it is higher in different places from echo to echo. The average SNR of these two echoes is 1.4 not 2. The SNR of a sequence is the $\sqrt{}$ (square root) of the number of nex.

> **Teaching Moment:** The number of NSAs (or nex, depending of your system manufacturer) is how many times a line is filled by **successive** TRs: 2 NSAs means line 1 is filled by the first and second TR, line 2 is filled by TR 3 and 4, line 3 by TR 5 and 6, etc. It is done this way to help lessen the effect of patient motion on IQ.

Scan Matrix

Phase and frequency have a huge effect on SNR, resolution, and scan time. Let's consider phase matrix first. What is the first thing you do to save time? Drop the phase matrix, right? Lowering the phase steps makes pixels larger, increasing SNR and decreasing scan time. Phase has no effect on image contrast.

Lowering the phase without lowering frequency makes the pixels anisotropic (not square) and can contribute to blur. A small drop in phase (256 down to 224) will not make a huge difference, but 256 down to 160 will.

Frequency Matrix

The frequency matrix will not affect scan time a great deal (just a little). It would not be my first choice to try to save time. A higher frequency matrix means the FEG is applied for longer (it has more work to do) than for a lower matrix (e.g. a 384 matrix vs. 192). Consequently, the TE pushes out by a ms or two and a longer TE may need longer TRs. Time goes up.

Just as with the phase, lowering the frequency matrix makes the pixels larger and less square, and can cause blurring while increasing SNR. Dropping the frequency matrix will also require the phase matrix to drop. Phase is always less than or equal to frequency. A few sequences will allow the phase matrix to be greater than the frequency matrix.

Frequency matrix can and will affect echo train balancing because it changes the minimum TE, echo spacing, and ultimately the ETL in terms of milliseconds. Remember to try to keep the pixels as square as possible.

The following scenario is one I have seen many times, and it can spiral out of control from blindly adjusting the frequency matrix and piling on other factors to correct for the previous one.

You need higher resolution on a sequence. You increase the frequency matrix to get smaller pixels, higher resolution, and not change scan time, right? The results are pixelly grainy images from low SNR and some blur from the anisotropic pixels. You add a nex to get more SNR, but to get a shorter scan time you increase the ETL, but need a longer TR and get more blur from the long ETL. The images are really no better, if not worse than what you started with. What gives? What has happened is that multiple factors added up to blurring, increased time, and maybe not good SNR. Here is a way of fixing a lack of resolution from a couple of different angles. You want a good balance between SNR, scan time, and resolution.

First, **square pixels are your friend**. See if your pixels are square. If not, make them square and run the sequence and take a look. For example, for a 256 × 384 matrix, split the difference and try 256 × 256. That may be all you need to do. Lowering the frequency to match the phase to square up the pixels will increase the SNR and lessen blur. If the SNR is increased, maybe drop a nex to save time. If you need more resolution, try 320 × 320. Change one thing at a time.

The next item to try in the fix is the ETL. Is it too long, too short? Adding to the ETL is not always the answer.

Echo Train Length

Know the consequence of your action.

The ETL is a user-controlled parameter used to shorten scan time. It is the number of echoes produced per TR. For T1, use an ETL of 2–3.

- T1: Short TR, short TE, and short ETL.
- T2: Long TR, long TE and long ETL.
- PD: Long TR, intermediate TE, and medium ETL. As previously stated, the new PD weighting, considered a "hybrid," is a long TR (2500–4000 ms), a longer TE (30–40 ms), and an ETL of 6–9. It is not the classic PD of old with a long TR and short TE. **Note**: On these hybrid PDs, some radiologists are very particular about TR, wanting no less than a 3500 ms. The reason for this is to remove as much T1 contrast as possible.

Considerations for ETL

- The longer the ETL, the more T2 you will add to the k-space, hence the need for a short ETL on T1s.
- Longer ETLs will add some blur to the images.
- The longer the ETL, the longer the TR needs to be. Again, watch the TR in T1 land.
- While the time saving is a boon, it needs to be used for good. Review Chapter 5 for additional information.
- Each echo comes from a 180° refocusing pulse, so SAR goes up on long ETLs.
- Blurring comes not only from the ETL, but from the time or "space" in between echoes (see next section, "Echo Spacing").

Echo Spacing

The echo spacing (ES) is the time in ms or "space" in between each echo in the train. The longer the space, the more blur you should expect. Also, the longer the ES, the further out the maximum TE will be, and the greater amount of the T2 by the end of the Echo Train. You will see in the next section, "Echo Train Balancing," that the minimum TE is also the ES. Parameters that affect TE also affect ES.

Consideration for ES: Anything affecting the time that the frequency encoding is applied **increases ES.**

Factors that Affect TE:

- Frequency FOV. **Small** vs. large.
- Frequency matrix. **High** vs. low.
- Receiver bandwidth. **Narrow** vs. wide.
- The longer the ES, the faster you get into T2 land, and the more blur you add to the images.
- Lastly, how good is your gradient system? If the gradients are not very fast, the ES (min TE) goes up.

The shorter the ES, the better the IQ. Remember ES only applies to multi-echo SE sequences, not GRE and conventional SE sequences. Even with the multi-echo GREs (also called MERGE or MEDIC sequences), the ES is of little consequence. The weighting on these is T2* with an ETL or number of echoes usually of 4 or 5, so echo train balancing and short ES is not a big concern.

Echo Train Balancing

What is echo train balancing? The echo train runs in time from the minimum TE (Min. TE) to the maximum TE (Max. TE). This time may be from 8–10 ms to 200 ms or more. Most manufacturers display this to you in one way or another. FSEs have two or more echoes. The shortest, or minimum TE, is the echo spacing (ES). Aim for a Min. TE of 10 ms or less. The shorter the better, and the less blur. With the Min and Max. TE displayed, if you multiply the ES (Min. TE) by the ETL, that will equal the Max. TE. What I mean by ET balancing is that you want your effective TE (ETE) in the middle of the ET. When I teach ET balancing, I only use it on ETLs of six or more. Balancing on T1s with two to three echoes is not worth the effort. For

T1s you want the Min. TE as your ETE and with only two or three echoes, there is not a whole lot to balance. What balancing does is put your |ETE in the middle of the train, which in turn puts the desired TEs into the center of *k*-space. **Think of the ETE as the fulcrum in a seesaw.** If the fulcrum is not in the middle, a seesaw does not work too well. There is some easy math needed to figure out the center of the ET. It is simple division and addition.

Figure 11.5 is an example of an ET running from 9.1 to 118.3 ms. With the ES (Min. TE) of 9.1 ms, and with an ETL of 13, that means the ET runs from 9.1 to 118.3. Here your effective TE is 91 ms. This ET is not balanced. To balance, you will need more echoes. You do not change your ETE as that is the image contrast you want.

What to do to balance: Double your ETE and add the minimum TE: 91 × 2 = 182, plus 9 = 191. From this math, you want the Max. TE to be 191 ms. **You need to lengthen the ETL to get Max. TE out to 191 ms.** So, add seven echoes. Let's do the math again: 9.1 ms × 20 echoes = 182 ms, + 9 ms = 191 ms. This math worked out perfectly. Your math may not. A millisecond or two either way is not a big deal.

The benefits from a combination of square pixels and echo train balancing are optimum image contrast and lessening blur from the long ETL. Some echo trains are unnecessarily long, causing higher SAR, increased blur, and sub-optimal image contrast. No image or protocol is perfect, but there is often room for improvement.

Optimization of any kind is a trial and error or hit and miss kind of process.

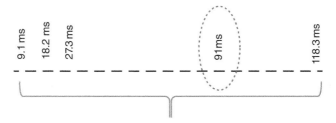

Figure 11.5 An unbalanced echo train.

Review: Double your effective TE, and add the minimum TE. That math value should be your Max. TE for the desired TE. So, in Figure 11.5, 91 × 2 = 182, + 9 = 191. To balance, you need to add echoes until the math works (Figure 11.6). **Do not change the ETE to make the math work, change the ETL to make the math work. That TE is your contrast.** Note that a millisecond or two either way is not a big deal; we are not going to Pluto. Sometimes the math comes out perfectly, other times not so. To make little changes to the echo spacing if you want the math spot on, adjust the receiver bandwidth. Narrowing it will increase the Min. TE and bump out the Max. TE and increase the SNR. Be careful not to narrow it too much, especially at 3 T, due to chemical shift artifact.

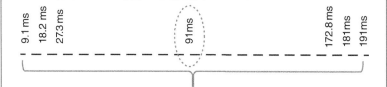

Figure 11.6 A balanced echo train. The ET has been adjusted to 20 so it now runs from 9.1 to 191 ms. ET spacing is still 9.1 ms. Effective TE is still 91 ms. Here is the math again: Double your effective TE and add the minimum ET: 91 × 2 = 182, now add 9 = 191. Max. TE needed is 191 ms. Again, a couple of ms either way with the above math is not a big deal. The unbalanced ET in Figure 11.5 was way off by 30 ms or more.

Slice Thickness and Slice Gap

Slice Thickness

A sequence's slice thickness needs to be appropriate for the anatomy being imaged. Thick slices of 6–8 mm are common for a liver, while 3 mm slices for internal auditory canals

(IACs) or pituitary studies are the norm. Logically, a high-resolution study has thin slices with a small gap in between them. Thick slices contribute to "partial volume effect." A small structure can hide within a thick slice. It is there, but you cannot see it.

Slice thickness is determined by two methods:

1. *The slope or steepness of the SSG* is adjusted for the required slice thickness. Figure 11.2 shows an example of how a steep or shallow gradient can change the FOV. It works the same for slice thickness. **Steep is a thin slice; shallow is a thick slice**.
2. *The transmitted RF bandwidth:* An RF pulse is not just one frequency, but many frequencies. It is a "range" of them. More frequencies transmitted equals a wide bandwidth for a thick slice or a narrow bandwidth for a thin slice.

Slice Gap

This represents an amount of tissue between slices that is not imaged. It is a percentage of the slice thickness. The different vendors state gap differently. Some state a percentage (%). Others let you enter a discrete gap. A 5 mm slice with a 0.5 gap means you scan 5 mm, then skip 2.5 mm or half the slice. A 0.5 gap is a big gap. Typical gaps are 0.10–0.20 (10–20%). A gap of 0.20 means scan 5 mm, skip 1 mm. Math: $5 \times 0.2(20\%) = 1.0$. Thin slices usually have no gap.

Fractional Echo

Fractional echo means you are not collecting the entire echo, only part of it (say 85% of it). This option is usually reserved for CE-MRAs to save time (TR). When you do not collect the entire echo, you will lose signal. This loss is offset by having gadolinium on board for the MRA. Around 99% of all sequences collect the entire echo. You want every little bit of signal you

Full Echo   Fractional Echo

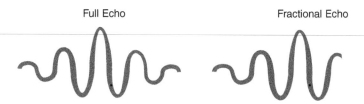

Figure 11.7 A fractional or partial echo, where only about three quarters of the echo is sampled. This is done for speed, a shorter TR.

can get. The added signal we get from having the gadolinium on board makes up for the signal loss from the partial echo. Figure 11.7 displays a full echo on the left, which is, say, 7 ms, but a fractional echo of 4 ms. The receiver is shut off during the echo. Those 3 ms can make a big difference in scan time during a CE-MRA time wise. Fractional echoes are also referred to as asymmetric echoes.

Bandwidth

Every sequence has two bandwidths (B/W): A **receiver** B/W and a little mentioned **transmitter** B/W.

Receiver Bandwidth

Vendors have different ways of expressing receiver bandwidth (rBW): GE expresses it as kHz, Siemens as Hz/Px (Hertz per pixel), and Philips as WFS (water–fat separation). This parameter has a direct influence on several things: SNR, chemical shift artifact, TE, and in an oblique way, the TR.

The best way to think of it is as "narrow or wide B/W."

You should know how to adjust the B/W on your system in order to gain a little signal or decrease chemical shift artifact. Sometimes you need to tweak the Min. TE for echo train balancing. The B/W is actually a sampling rate: Basically, how fast or slow is the echo sampled. Think of the receiver B/W as miles per hour. A wide B/W is a faster sampling rate (say 60 mph) while a narrow B/W is a slower sampling rate (30 mph).

You can also think of it this way. The echo needs sampling a certain number of times. Do you sample at 60 mph and finish quickly, or at 30 mph and take longer? There are of course trade-offs with the receiver B/W.

- *GE:* **kHz**: Represents the number of Hertz **across the FOV** in the **frequency direction**. A large number of Hertz is a wide B/W. It allows more Hz (frequencies) in a pixel: Chemical shift artifact, lower Min. TE, lower SNR. It is a fast sampling rate.
- *Siemens:* **Hz/Px**: is a straightforward interpretation. High Hx/Px means more frequencies per pixel (same as GE) so less chemical shift, a lower SNR. It is a fast sampling rate.
- *GE + Siemens:* Increasing the kHz or Hz/Px is a **wider** B/W.
- *Philips:* **Water–Fat Shift**: A low WFS means more frequencies per pixel, less chemical shift artifact, and a shorter Min. TE. A small WFS is a fast sampling rate. WFS is stated in mm or how large the artifact will be. It is nice to be told how big your chemical shift artifact will be. For example, a 1.4 mm WFS when scanning 0.7 mm pixels means your artifact will be 2 pixels wide.

Earlier I suggested thinking of the B/W as a sampling rate or speed. A wide B/W, being a fast sampling rate, results in a shorter minimum TE. The opposite of course is true: A narrow B/W is slower, causing a longer Min. TE with higher SNR but with more chemical shift.

What else does a longer TE do to you? **It increases your echo spacing, which in turn can cause blurring.** It may also, on occasion, cause you to have to increase your TR. Remember, the TE lives within the TR, and TR is a **finite** amount of time to do the work. Increasing the Min. TE uses up more of the TR and you may not fit all the slices into the TR, so you may have to increase it a little.

Wide versus Narrow Receiver Bandwidth

A **wide receiver B/W** samples everything, including the ends of the echo where SNR is not very good (Figure 11.8). If you average out the good and bad from a wide B/W, the overall SNR is lower than if only getting the good stuff from a narrow B/W.

A **narrow receiver B/W** samples just the center of the echo where the signal amplitude is highest compared to a relatively low-level noise. Where there is a high amount of signal over hopefully a low amount of noise then the SNR is very good.

Figure 11.8 shows the differences between narrow and wide receiver B/W. All scan factors being the same, a narrow B/W has a higher SNR when compared to a wide B/W. Do not try to

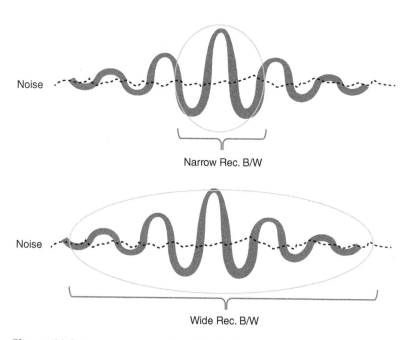

Figure 11.8 In a narrow receiver B/W only the "sweet spot" (circled) of the echo is sampled. In a wide receiver B/W the entire echo is sampled (circled) including the lower SNR portions (at the beginning and end of the echo).

memorize the details for both. Remember one and the opposite is true of the other.

> *Wide:* Shorter Min. TE, ↓ SNR, ↓ chemical shift, ↓ blur, ↓ ES.
> *Narrow:* Long Min. TE, ↑ SNR, ↑ chemical shift, ↑ blur, ↑ ES.

- On T1s, a wide B/W is common, making the TE shorter.
- On T2s, a narrow B/W helps to increase SNR, especially on the late echoes of the ET where SNR is at a premium.
- Always use a wide B/W scanning on 3 T to decrease chemical shift.

Teaching Moment: On high resolution sequences, use as wide a B/W as possible to decrease blur. A wide B/W = short echo spacing, and short echo spacing = less blur. Chemical shift artifact and blur may obscure anatomy/pathology.

Transmitter Bandwidth

Transmitter B/W is one way to change slice thickness. A wider transmitter B/W produces a thicker slice, with the opposite being true – a narrow transmitter B/W gives a thinner slice. Transmitter is explained in more detail later in this chapter.

An RF pulse is just not a single frequency (e.g. 63 MHz), but rather a range of frequencies or a "bandwidth." For example, a bandwidth expressed as 63 ± 5 MHz describes a group of radiofrequencies with a center frequency of 63, with 5 less than 63 and 5 greater than 63. So, this band or range of frequencies runs from 58 to 68 Mhz. Tissues precessing from 63 ± 5 MHz are a slice and will be excited when exposed to this RF pulse. One side of the slice is at 58 MHz, and the other side of the slice is at 68 MHz because of its position along the SSG (Figure 11.9).

The second way to alter slice thickness is to change the amplitude or steepness of the SSG (Figure 11.10). This is the

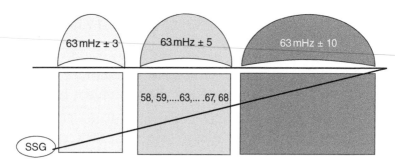

Figure 11.9 Three different transmitter B/Ws, all with the same center frequency of 63mHz, exciting three different slice thicknesses. SSG is constant, while transmitter B/W is varied.

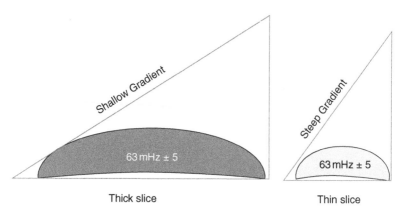

Figure 11.10 A low and high amplitude SSG with the same B/W (63 ± 5) as in Figure 11.9. A steeper SSG yields a thinner slice.

same principle as the FEG. A steep or high amplitude SSG will cause a thin slice, shallow or low amplitude a thick slice. **In a high amplitude application, the same frequency B/W is crunched into less of an area.** The opposite is also true.

Which one does your scanner use? The answer is that more than likely it will be changing the SSG. Why? **Applying a gradient is more time efficient than RF.**

Speaking of transmitted RF, the RF pulse applied for slice selection or refocusing is represented as B_1. What is seldom, if ever, mentioned is that the 90° and 180° are **not** pulses with a flip angle embedded into them but a timing aspect. The RF pulse is applied long enough to change the angle of the longitudinal

NMV to say 90°, or twice as long for a 180°. A partial flip angle is a quick "blip" of RF in order to achieve the desired flip angle. Partial flip angles apply mostly to GREs.

Rectangular (Rec.) FOV

Rectangular FOV, phase FOV, or partial FOV is an option to shorten scan time. The FOV is always square unless this option is applied. A Rec. FOV does not scan the entire FOV in the phase direction. A general rule in MR is to have phase in the short axis of the patient so that you can shorten the scan time. In Figure 11.11, the frequency direction is S/I and

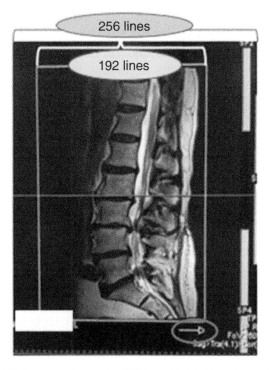

Figure 11.11 Shows rectangular FOV applied in the phase direction (circled). Scan time drops by one quarter. The scan matrix was set to 256 × 256 but a three-quarter Rec. FOV was applied to the FOV in phase direction, so 192 lines of phase were scanned, not 256. **Resolution is maintained, as the matrix is not altered.**

phase is A/P. The FOV needs to be large enough to cover S/I, but that makes it too big in the A/P. Why scan air? The reason for "shortening up the phase direction" is to save time. Scanning lines of phase costs time, so scanning fewer lines means a shorter scan time (see section "Scan Time Equations" in Chapter 14). The amount of Rec. FOV can be changed. This time savings, of course, and as usual, come at a price, that of decreased SNR. **Rec. FOV does not affect resolution**; for example, with a 256 × 256 matrix, when a three-quarter Rec. FOV is applied, only three quarters of the lines in the phase direction are scanned, and time drops by one quarter. Rec. FOV does not change the scan matrix, it just scans fewer phase lines.

Let me explain the "short axis" and its relation to the phase direction. As I have already said, the FOV is square. Sometimes you need a bigger FOV to cover the anatomy in **one direction** but that means the FOV is now too big in the other. An example of this is in the brain. We are all mostly "narrower" R/L and "longer" A/P. The FOV needs to be big enough to cover the A/P direction, causing extra FOV R/L. There is no need to scan air as it adds nothing to the image except a longer scan time. There are exceptions, for example sagittals in the spine, where logic dictates to run phase A/P to save time. That is how it used to be years ago. The problem with that is motion. Motion runs A/P (phase direction) and obscures the spinal cord. An anterior saturation pulse does not always work well. Nowadays, phase and frequency are usually swapped so that phase is S/I (long axis) with no phase wrap or phase oversampling turned on. This way motion runs S/I and is seen anterior to the spine.

Swapping phase and frequency directions swaps the directions. If doing axials in the brain, if phase is R/L then frequency is A/P. Swapping makes phase A/P and frequency R/L. Swapping is a nice option, but do not forget that wrap is always in the phase direction so watch where the long/ short axis falls. We have all been a victim of wrap from swapping P/F.

> **Teaching Moment:** Older systems had both no phase wrap and Rec. FOV options but did not allow for simultaneous usage. It was one or the other. Now software improvements allow for use of them at the same time.

No Phase Wrap/Phase Oversampling/ Fold-Over Suppression

We have all experienced the wrap artifact. Wrap happens when you have tissue outside of the FOV in the phase direction. What happens if you cannot have phase in the short axis? This can happen with very small FOVs in high resolution studies.

When you need small FOVs as in pituitary, IAC, or prostate, wrap is inevitable. The anti-aliasing options – no phase wrap or phase oversampling – are your friends.

Phase oversampling scans extra lines of phase eliminating or minimizing wrap (Figure 11.12). It will increase both scan time and SNR. These extra lines of phase are scanned at a lower resolution and are then discarded so are not displayed in the final image.

No phase wrap (NPW) doubles the entire FOV, doubles the matrix, and halves the nex. The images show no wrap, and both resolution and SNR are maintained. NPW happens in the background. More information on artifact control is provided in Chapter 12.

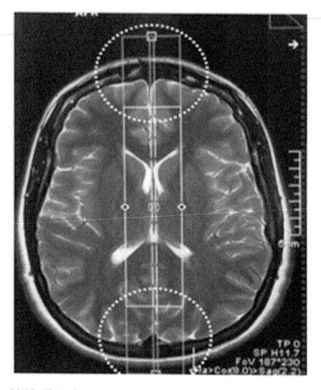

Figure 11.12 This shows the area being "over-sampled" (circled), removing wrap.

Teaching Moment: Wrap does not only happen in the phase direction. It can happen in the slice direction as well on 3Ds (Figure 11.13). There is an option to oversample in the slice select direction. Extra slices are sampled in the slice direction and then are discarded, removing slice wrap. Scan time does increase with this option.

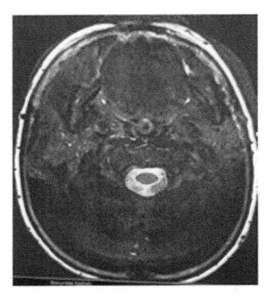

Figure 11.13 Slice wrap, seen on 3D sequences. The base of the skull anatomy is clearly visible, wrapping superiorly on this T2 weighted 3D sequence.

Scan parameter review: Do not just blindly start changing parameters. **Know the consequences of your actions.** All factors affect one or more of the IQ triangle considerations.

Square pixels are your friend in 2D and isotropic voxels in 3D. Balance that echo train for optimum image contrast. The desired image contrast should be in the middle of the ET. Keep the ES short for less blur. Do not scan a higher frequency just to get more resolution. In theory it works, but it has a ripple effect on IQ as the frequency matrix affects multiple other factors.

Find the balance between SNR, resolution, and scan time. This is a trial and error project. There is no magic formula. Nothing is free in MRI. Everything costs you something, somewhere, somehow. The geometric parameters, SNR and resolution, are the next two areas in the image IQ triangle (see Figure 11.1).

Concatenations or Acquisitions

I was unsure which chapter to include this concept in, but I certainly could not leave it out. The terms are very often confused, confusing, and/or misunderstood.

First, the terminology is confusing because it is used differently by different vendors, as in receiver bandwidth: GE and Hitachi use "acquisitions," while Siemens uses "concatenations." Next is the concept of it. The basic reason to have one or two or even three acquisitions is either to make breath-holds shorter, or to lower the minimum TR on a sequence. When you increase the number of acquisitions, you are going to do multiple measurements over multiple TRs, called "multi-slice imaging."

Here is an example of when to increase your acquisitions. You need **30** slices of coverage on a T1 weighted sequence, but that coverage makes your minimum TR 1010 ms. You have two options. You could do two sequences of 15 slices each with overlapping coverage, or increase your acquisitions from 1 to 2. This option lets you halve the TR to 505 ms, which keeps you in T1 land and the sequences are together, not separate. The scanner will do half the slices (**15**) with 505 TR in the first acquisition then the other **15** slices with another 505 TR in the second acquisition. This is a single sequence, not two separate ones, as stated earlier. T1 image contrast is maintained.

Another example of when to increase acquisitions is when you are running a T2 weighted breath-hold sequence with a scan time of, say, 1:15 s (75 s). Your acquisitions are set at 2. Here comes the math: 75 s ÷ 2 acquisitions = a 37 s breath-hold. A reasonable breath-hold for your patient is 20 s. That 37 s breath-hold will not work. If you increase the acquisitions to 3, then the breath-holds become 25 s, still not good enough. Raise the acquisitions to 4, and the breath-holds are now 18 s. IQ should be good as that is a reasonable breath-hold for many people.

Increasing the acquisitions is a way to shorten the scan time without adversely affecting image contrast from either using too high a TR, decreasing the nex, lowering the phase matrix, or increasing the amount of phase FOV.

A minor drawback of using more than one acquisition is that if the patient moves during the sequence, or if the breath-holds are not the same, you will notice that the images may shift a little bit from image to image. That is because the anatomy is in a slightly different place from acquisition to acquisition. This occurrence is a problem on axial breath-holds in the abdomen. If the patient does not hold their breath the same way each time, the anatomy will be at different places for each acquisition and you could miss tissue. If there is an option to acquire the breath-hold slices in **sequential order**, this is a good choice here.

Sequential Order Acquisition

A sequential order acquisition means that the scanner will image/acquire the slices in their sequential order. What I mean by this is that if you have 21 slices, the scanner will acquire the slices in order: 1–7 in one breath-hold, then 8–14 on the next breath-hold, and finally 15–21 for the last breath-hold. This option can decrease the possibility of missing too much tissue. You may miss tissue between slices 7 and 8, then 14 and 15. The system can acquire in either ascending (1, 2, 3, 4) or descending (5, 4, 3, 2, 1) order.

Notes

12 Image Artifacts

Chapter at a Glance

Motion
   Motion Suppression Sequences
Flow Artifact/Phase Mis-registration
   Flow Comp or GMR
RF Artifacts
Wrap/Aliasing/Fold-over Artifact
Gibbs Artifact (Ringing/Truncation)
Chemical Shift Artifact
   Chemical Shift: Bandwidth
   Chemical Shift of the Second Kind
Cross-talk
   Control of Cross-talk
Cross-excitation
Gradient Warp or Distortion
Metal Artifacts
Corduroy Artifact
Annifact

MRI Physics: Tech to Tech Explanations, First Edition. Stephen J. Powers.
© 2021 John Wiley & Sons Ltd. Published 2021 by John Wiley & Sons Ltd.

Moiré Fringe Artifact or Zebra Artifact
Magnetic Susceptibility Artifact
Dielectric Effect or Standing Wave
Magic Angle Artifact

An artifact is basically unwanted signal(s) that does not contribute to or detracts from IQ. Artifacts are a daily occurrence in MR. Artifacts become worse when the SNR of a sequence is low. Artifacts can be grouped into three main causes: Hardware, physics, and data sampling.

Let me start out with this. Every image has artifact(s) somewhere, somehow, for some reason. No image is perfect. We can only hope to minimize the impact of artifacts on IQ.

Motion

Motion is the most common and detrimental artifact going. Here we are talking gross patient motion, where everything is moving. Motion is always seen in the phase direction. There are multiple simple ways to combat motion, including patient comfort, coaching, immobilization, saturation pulses, and motion suppression sequences.

- **Comfort.** Provide an extra pad, a blanket (careful at 3 T), or cushions under the knees.
- **Coaching.** Tell the patient what is needed for a good exam, and go over the breathing instructions prior to the exam.
- **Immobilize** with pads or straps.

These only take a few minutes and do make a difference. Even a good patient can only be good for so long. The pulse sequence itself can make a difference to the artifact: Long TR/TE vs. short TR/TE. DWIs and IRs are extremely motion sensitive.

Why Is Motion Only Seen in the Phase Direction?:
The answer is pretty simple. First, I shall explain slice and
frequency directions. Both frequency and slice encoding
take less than a millisecond to perform. Phase encoding is
a different story. The phase encoding happens in between
excitation and refocusing; the echo is sampled multiple
ms later. There is a time delay from phase encoding to the
TE (Figures 12.1 and 12.2). From phase encoding to TE is
really three quarters of the TE. If the TE is say 100 ms, the
time from phase encode to the TE is 75 ms.

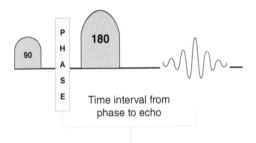

Figure 12.1 Note the time interval from phase encoding to the
TE in SE. This time interval, repeated many times over during
the scan, causes motion to "smear" in the phase direction.

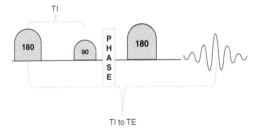

Figure 12.2 Note the time interval from the Inversion Pulse
to the TE in IR. This time interval, repeated many times over
during the scan, also causes motion to "smear" in the phase
direction.

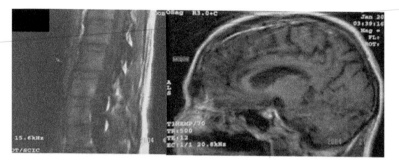

Figure 12.3 Motion artifact in phase direction on lumbar spine and sagittal brain scans.

When a patient moves, the phase encoding applied to a tissue at position "A" is not in the same position at TE, it is in position "B." This manifests as ghosting/blurring **in the phase direction** (Figure 12.3). Motion is worse in long TR/TE sequences. STIR/FLAIR sequences are highly susceptible to motion. There is a time interval between the IR pulse and the TE – a big one.

Also, phase encoding is repeated many times over many TRs, so tissues have multiple opportunities to be in various locations over time.

Besides the motion prevention methods already discussed, there are sequences designed to greatly decrease motion artifact. A generic description of these sequences is "non-Cartesian" or radial k-space filling. The vendor names are: Propeller (GE), BLADE (Siemens), Multi-Vane (Philips), Jet (Toshiba), and RADAR (Hitachi). These sequences work very well. Areas where these are particularly useful are the uterus, liver/kidneys, and prostate. In the abdomen/pelvis, couple these with respiratory triggering and you can achieve double the motion suppression but at the expense of time.

Motion Suppression Sequences

These sequences work by filling k-space in a rotating section of lines in a radial pattern. Think of how an airplane's propeller

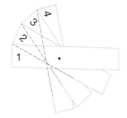

Figure 12.4 The motion suppression technique. Sections of *k*-space are sampled, and then rotated with some overlap. Overlap is the key to motion suppression.

rotates. Groups of lines of *k*-space are rotated on a central point or axis (Figure 12.4). A group of, say, 20 lines is rotated and overlaps by, say, 10 lines with the previous group or "blade." It is the overlap that decreases the motion. Blade 1 is scanned, followed blade 2. Blade 2 is compared to blade 1, and pixels that match between them stay in *k*-space, whereas pixels that do not match are thrown out. Motion causes the pixels from blade to blade not to match up. Blade 3 is then scanned, compared to blade2, bad pixels are removed, then blade 4 is scanned. See a pattern developing? Non-matching pixels (motion) are removed section by section.

FYIs on Motion Suppression Sequences:

- They do not necessarily have a shorter scan time as they are FSEs.
- Have increased SNR as the center of *k*-space is constantly being sampled.
- Can be fat-sat, T1, T2, PD, or FLAIR weighted.
- Can be run post IV contrast.
- Can be respiratory triggered.
- Work best for "in-plane" motion.
- Some radiologists find them "flat" when compared to regular FSEs.
- Are FSE based sequences.

What about just scanning fast? That is an option, but as usual, everything costs you something somewhere in MR. That cost is in either SNR or resolution, or both. Here is a list on how to scan faster:

- **Drop a nex:** Lowers scan time but loses SNR.
- **Lower the phase:** Lower resolution (pixels bigger and not square).
- **Lower the TR:** Low SNR if TR too low: Watch your T2 weighting.
- **Use Rec. FOV:** Lowers SNR with wrap possible.
- **Increase ETL:** Can increase blur and take you out of T1 land.
- **Increase parallel imaging:** Loses SNR and some resolution.
- **Delete Sat Pulses:** Allows a lower TR and may increase motion.

Know the consequences of your actions. Everything, and I mean everything, affects something somewhere in MRI. Often it affects more than one of the IQ triangle's items.

Flow Artifact/Phase Mis-registration

Pulsatile artifacts are really nothing more than motion. However, rather than gross patient motion, only a very small part of the anatomy is moving. It just happens to be due to the flow of blood. Moving blood (protons) traveling through a gradient picks up phase. Different phases within the slice look like motion and are projected in the **phase** direction. There are three ways to deal with flow artifacts: **Flow compensation (flow comp), saturation pulses, and swap phase and frequency.** Saturation pulses will increase SAR and possibly scan time as this is extra work the scanner has to do, so a longer TR may be needed. Flow comp is a set of gradient pulses that help to lessen the phase changes caused by moving blood in a vessel. **As a general rule,**

long TR and TE sequences should have flow comp/gradient motion refocusing (GMR) applied. This extra work increases the TE and likely the TR. It is extra work being done by the scanner.

Flow Comp or GMR

This is a pair of equal and opposite polarity gradients, a gradient reversal technique if you like. Remember that in DWI, moving protons in a gradient pick up phase. You want that in DWI, but not in regular imaging. If you turn on an equal and opposite polarity gradient (Figure 12.5) you will correct the effects of the first gradient. Flow comp happens prior to the TE, so an increase in TE when flow comp is turned on can be expected. Remember that any extra work you want the scanner to do will cost you somewhere, whether it is with a longer TR or TE (Figure 12.6).

Flow comp is not only a motion suppression technique; it can also be used to make flow bright. Your TOF MRA sequences have or should have flow comp turned on. Yes, it is TOF and flow should be bright next to the saturated background, but every little bit helps for increased signal and less artifact. Flow comp should also be turned on for T2 and STIRs in the spine as well. Radiologists want bright CSF and a dark cord. Flow comp helps with that. As stated earlier in the book, if you are running sagittal spines with phase S/I and with sat pulses also S/I, lose

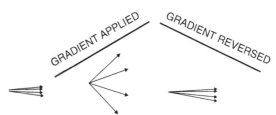

Protons in-phase   Protons lose phase   Protons re-phased

Figure 12.5 The effects of gradient reversal on protons de-phased by the first gradient, then the re-phasing effect of the equal and opposite gradient field.

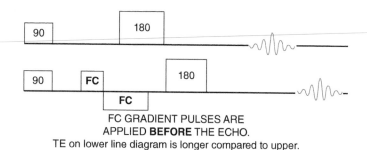

FC GRADIENT PULSES ARE
APPLIED **BEFORE** THE ECHO.
TE on lower line diagram is longer compared to upper.

Figure 12.6 Two PSDs without and with flow comp. The TE lengthens due to the extra gradient applications. More work equals more time.

the sats. They are basically working against flow comp. Think about it, flow comp is on to brighten up CSF; it is flowing S/I – slowly, but flowing. That flow takes it through a sat pulse just like an MRA saturating out venous blood on carotid images. S/I sats result in CSF being slightly darker; flow comp makes it slightly brighter. Opposites.

But you have the sats on to prevent wrap. This is not an issue if you have anti-wrap techniques turned on. You do not need both. All the sats do is add to the patient's SAR and lengthen your TR. Delete them.

What about flow comp and T1s? Yes and no. **Yes,** for post gadolinium in the brain. It helps a little with pulsatile motion. **No,** for pre gadolinium in the brain. **Applying flow comp pre gadolinium can make the vessels bright as if you have given gadolinium even though you have not. It also increases the TE and may lose T1 contrast.**

Flow Comp for Long TR Sequences

Flow comp decreases pulsatile artifacts (phase mis-registration) on long TR sequences (Figure 12.7). Long TR/TE sequences without flow comp allow moving spins to de-phase, causing an artifact. Short TR/TE sequences are kind of "self-flow comp'd". Short TR/TEs do not allow for much pulsatile phase mis-registration artifact.

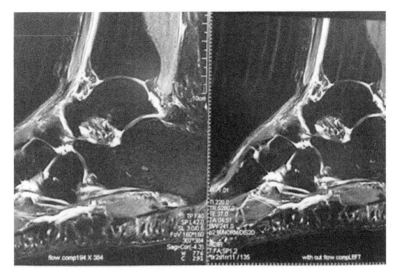

Figure 12.7 Two sagittal ankle STIR images, the right scanned without flow comp and the left scanned with flow comp. Note lessening of pulsatile flow artifact due to flow comp.

RF Artifacts

MR uses RF pulses for excitation and refocusing. We need to keep our RF in the room, and outside RF out. This is done with an RF shielded room or Faraday cage. The Faraday cage is akin to lead shielding in an x-ray room. When unwanted RF either gets into the room or is generated within the room the coil may see it, it gets put into k-space, and we get an artifact (Figure 12.8). All signals have to go somewhere in k-space.

Wrap/Aliasing/Fold-over Artifact

We have all seen this artifact. No MRI tech in the world has not gotten wrap. Wrap comes from having tissue outside the FOV in the phase direction. Basically, that tissue is not sampled

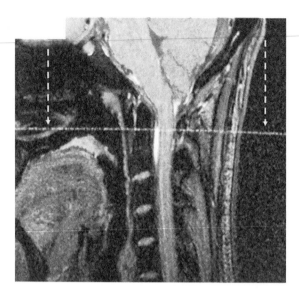

Figure 12.8 RF artifact or zipper (dotted lines) from opening the scan room door while scanning. This is considered a **narrow** B/W (only a few frequencies) leak seen in the phase direction. Its position in the phase direction depends on its frequency. A **wide** B/W leak has many zippers and is also seen in the frequency direction.

enough (it is under sampled) and the tissue is mapped on the wrong side of the FOV. **Under sampled** means there are insufficient data to know exactly where the signal should go in k-space (an incomplete address as it were). For example, the left side gets put on the right, and the right side gets put on the left.

Sampling of a signal (in MR, the echo) is governed by the **Nyquist theorem**. The Nyquist theorem states that a sine wave needs to be sampled at twice its frequency to get an accurate measurement. So, if a wave's frequency is 50, it needs to be sampled 100 times. In the artifact "wrap," tissue outside the FOV in the phase direction is not sampled enough to satisfy the Nyquist theorem and that tissue's signal will be put in the wrong place in the image.

Figure 12.9 shows an example of the Nyquist theorem.

Wrap comes from having tissue outside the FOV in the phase direction. The scan matrix is applied only to the tissue **inside** the FOV, not outside. Tissue outside the FOV is not sampled enough. It does receive RF, even though you do not want to see it. If it gets RF, it will give signal, and those signals need to go somewhere. **Remember, RF is round or oval,** it is not square like we think. It extends outside of the FOV, and when tissue is outside the FOV, wrap happens. Accurate sampling is limited to tissue inside the FOV. Tissue outside the FOV gets under sampled and misplaced in *k*-space (Figure 12.10).

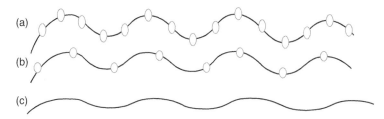

Figure 12.9 Sine wave A is sampled according to the Nyquist theorem, which will give an accurate depiction of the wave. In B, sine wave A is under sampled and will not give an accurate depiction of the wave, which will be seen as line C.

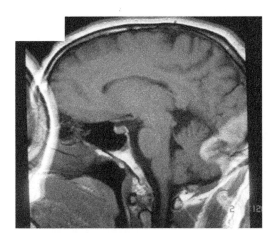

Figure 12.10 The anterior aspect of the face is under sampled and displaced posteriorly. The occipital area placed anteriorly.

Teaching Moment for Wrap: Here is a trouble shooting technique if you see a subtle area in the anatomy and question if it is an artifact or if it is real. A quick, cheap, and easy way to figure it out is to run the same sequence in a different plane. **Keep the same weighting. Do not change two variables.** If you see the same thing in the same place in another plane, it is real. If it has gone, it was an artifact. You can also just as easily swap phase or frequency. If it is an artifact, its position will change or it will disappear. If it stays, it is a real finding.

Gibbs Artifact (Ringing/Truncation)

The terms Gibbs, ringing, and truncation are often used interchangeably. The artifact occurs for several reasons:

1. *The pixels are not square,* meaning a large difference between phase and frequency matrix. When the phase matrix is half or less than half the frequency matrix, the less square the pixels will be. The less square the pixels, the worse the truncation artifact (Figure 12.11).
2. *High tissue contrast interfaces.* Bright tissue is next to dark tissue (Figure 12.12). In spine images there is high signal CSF and dark cord.

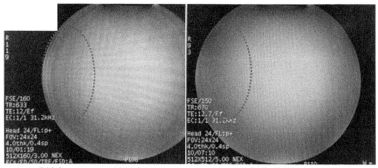

512 frequency × 160 phase.   515×512

Figure 12.11 Gibbs/Truncation artifact, cause 1: Anisotropic pixels on the left, and isotropic pixels on the right. Note the matrices for each.

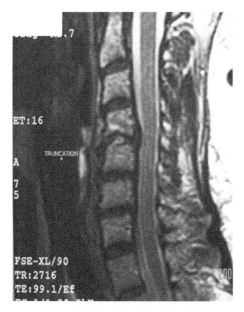

Figure 12.12 Gibbs/Truncation artifact, cause 2: Seen at high tissue contrast interfaces (cord and CSF). Looks like "zebra stripes" across the cord.

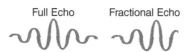

Figure 12.13 Gibbs/Truncation artifact, cause 3: Asymmetric echo. Only part of the echo is sampled. Fourier transform does not like the "cut-off" (or truncation). It would much prefer that the echo fade away to nothing.

3. **Partial or asymmetric echo acquisitions** if the entire echo is not sampled. Some CE-MRA sequences do this (Figure 12.13).

4. **FSE/TSE sequences.** SNR varies from echo to echo within *k*-space. Fourier transform does not like that (Figures 12.14 and 12.15).

If you are saying to yourself, "All these artifacts look the same," you are right, they do. Ringing, truncation, and Gibbs are all interchangeable terms because the artifacts look much the same. They will always be there, just more or less visible due to pixel size.

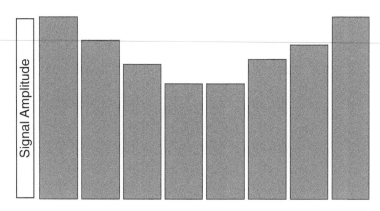

SNR varies from line to line in *k*-space

Figure 12.14 Gibbs/Truncation artifact, cause 4: Varying SNR from line to line in *k*-space in an FSE sequence can cause "ringing". Again, Fourier transform does not like signal variations.

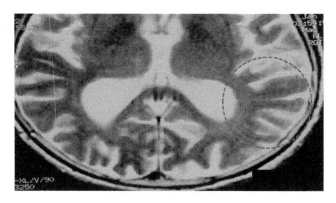

Figure 12.15 Gibbs/Truncation artifact, cause 4: Image windowed to demonstrate a ringing artifact (circled) on this T2 axial of the brain that comes from amplitude variations of echoes that can occur during an FSE.

Teaching Moment: These artifacts have various causes with similar fixes: That fix is **pixel size.** If the pixels are square and small, then ringing, Gibbs, and truncation for the most part will be minimized.

Chemical Shift Artifact

Chemical shift means that there is a difference or "shift" of PF between two substances or chemicals. Those substances are fat and water. Both these chemicals have different PFs, as was discussed in Chapter 6. We take advantage of that difference during a fat-sat sequence, but these same differences can also cause an artifact called chemical shift, or just chem shift. Chem shift is seen in the **frequency direction. The chem shift artifact has two different forms.** You see them both all the time. Chemical shift of the first kind is the most common. The cool kids call it "chem shift". The second kind you know as the out of phase (OOP) echo in an adrenal study. **The first kind you want to minimize, and the second kind you want to see.**

- Chemical shift of the first kind is affected/controlled by the receiver bandwidth (B/W) and is seen in one direction: Frequency.
- Chemical shift of the second kind is what you want when doing abdominal studies and is controlled by the TEs. It is seen in two directions, both phase and frequency. On an OOP TE it is a black line around the abdominal organs in **two directions: phase and frequency.** It is occasionally called or described as the "India ink" artifact.

Remember: Artifact in **one** direction = chem shift of **the first kind**.
Artifact in **two** directions = chem shift of **the second kind**.

Chemical Shift: Bandwidth

The receiver B/W defines the number of frequencies or Hz in each pixel. FOV also contributes to the artifact but I will not cover this now. As already stated, fat and water have different PFs and at higher field strengths the difference increases. This is a common concern at 3 T. You may have manually tuned for fat-sat at some time. What you are looking at is a spectrum of the frequencies of fat and water. There is some math involved. To get the frequency difference of fat and water, at 1.5 T multiply 3.5 ppm × 63.86 MHz = 224 Hz, and at 3 T 3.5 ppm × 127, = 440 Hz. Now, if you have a pixel that can hold 224 Hz or 440 Hz, great, no chemical shift. Everybody is happy. This scenario seldom if ever happens. Often you have too many frequencies that need to be put into a pixel. You can only put 5 pounds of something into a 5-pound bag. Put in 7 pounds and it oozes out. That ooze is chemical shift artifact (Figure 12.16). A narrow B/W puts more frequencies into a pixel, and if that number of frequencies exceeds the maximum then something is going to give. Here is an analogy:

- A bottle contains oil and water: Oil on top, water on the bottom. They separate and that is chemical shift.
- The bottle only holds so much. Keep adding either water or oil or both and have the paper towels ready.
- The same thing happens to a pixel: Fat on one side, water on the other. Too many frequencies and they spill out.
- If you add more oil to the bottle by using a narrow B/W, eventually the oil and water will spill out. Fat and water do that in a pixel.

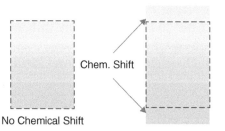
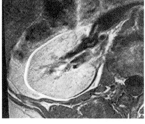

No Chemical Shift

Chem. Shift

Figure 12.16 Pixels are the dotted line. On the left, the pixel can hold all the frequencies and there is no chem shift. On the right, too many frequencies are put in the pixel and they ooze out. This is chem shift. In the axial image to the right, note the white line on the left aspect of the kidney and the dark line on the right. That is chem shift.

Chem shift is seen as a dark line on one side and a bright line on the other **in the frequency direction**. Why in the frequency direction? There are too many **frequencies** going into the pixels so naturally it is a **frequency direction artifact**. There are a few remedies for chem shift:

1. *Widen the B/W*, but this will decrease SNR.
2. *Swap phase and frequency.* This makes the artifact go in a different direction. It is still there, just in the A/P vs. R/L.
3. *Use fat-sat* if possible. It makes the whole fat/water oozing out thing go away, **but** you have just changed the image contrast and the radiologist may not want a fat-sat sequence.

Look at Figure 12.17. What else is there to note about the IQ on T1 sagittal L/S spine images? These are 3 T images, same slice and patient. Compare the right and left images.

- The narrow B/W on the right gives a higher SNR, but more blur from a larger echo spacing. Even with an ETL of 3, assuming a Min. TE of 12, the final echo is at 36 ms. It is not really T1.
- T1 contrast has also suffered. CSF has brightened significantly from the longer minimum TE on the right.
- Look at the area directly posterior to the vertebral bodies on the narrow B/W image on the right. Small herniations at L4/5 and L5/S1 are harder to see (circled).

I do not want to repeat too much, but here is yet another way to visualize how receiver B/W causes chem shift artifact. Figure 12.18 shows two identical spectrums of fat and water seen when performing manual tuning for fat-sat. In this example, water is the left peak, fat is on the right. The dotted square represents a pixel that we can put frequencies into by virtue of the chosen receiver B/W. On the left, the B/W is wide and "covers" or includes both peaks so no chem shift artifact

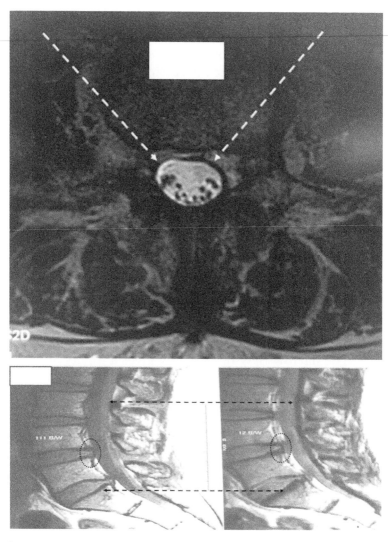

Figure 12.17 Both sets of images are windowed to demonstrate chem shift artifacts. Axial L/S spine artifact is R/L. Sagittal L/S spine shows the effect of wide and narrow B/W on chem shift.

will be seen. The B/W on the right is narrow and does not "cover" or include both peaks. There will be chem shift artifact. The dotted square is a 5-pound bag (a pixel). The wide B/W puts 5 pounds of frequencies into a 5-pound pixel, but the

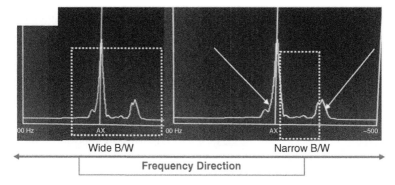

Wide B/W		Narrow B/W

Frequency Direction

Figure 12.18 Two images of a fat-sat tuning spectrum. **Wide receiver B/W** on the left lets the fat/water frequencies fit into the pixel. **Narrow receiver B/W** on the right caused the fat/water frequencies to not fit into the pixel. Chem shift artifact results as noted by arrows.

narrow B/W is trying to put 10 pounds of frequencies into a 5-pound pixel. The concept of receiver B/W can be a difficult one to understand, and when you add in the effects of it on IQ it can be daunting. Receiver B/W is a factor you do need to understand, especially on a 3 T.

Teaching Moment: General rules of thumb when working at 3 T. To achieve good IQ use: Wide receiver B/Ws, a high matrix (square pixels preferred), and finally 1– 3 nex.

Chemical Shift of the Second Kind

Look at Figure 12.19. What else do you see in the IP and OOP images?

Muscle and bone marrow are significantly darker. Fat has darkened somewhat. This is something that the radiologists look for in the adrenal glands. Adenomas and metastases have different appearances on IP vs. OOP.

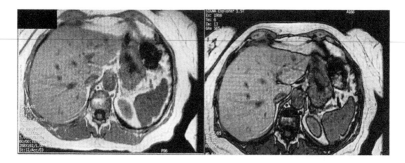

Figure 12.19 IP (left) and OOP (right) echoes in the abdomen. The OOP on the right is sometimes called chemical shift of the **second** kind. Note that this "chemical shift artifact" is seen in **two** directions, whereas the "regular" chem shift artifact is only seen in one direction (frequency) (see Figures 12.16 and 12.17).

> **Teaching Moment:** Do you ever see chemical shift of the second kind on anything but a GRE sequence? The answer is no, and this is why: **Because GREs have no 180° but a SE/FSE does.** As previously stated, the 180°'s job is to put the protons back into phase at the TE. So, even if the TE is an OOP TE in milliseconds, the protons will be in phase at TE and you will not see the canceling out effect of the opposed phase protons like you do on a GRE. Protons will never be OOP in a SE. Review Chapter 6 for more information on IP and OOP echoes.

Cross-talk

There are two kinds of cross-talk. One you see all the time and it is obvious; the other is much more subtle. Textbook cross-talk (the subtle one) happens when excitation pulses of adjacent slices have some RF in common. What I mean is, slice 1's excitation pulse profile has a few frequencies that are also in slice 2's. RF pulse is not a discrete or single number. Nor is an RF pulse square. It is actually a range or group of frequencies called a bandwidth (B/W) and is round. We think of RF pulses or our "slices" as square like a slice of bread but they are not.

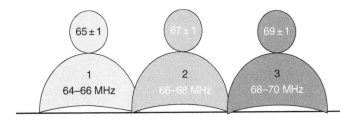

Figure 12.20 Adjacent slices that have frequencies in common can interfere with or "cross-talk" each other. The left slice has one frequency in common with the middle, and the middle has one frequency in common with the right. Signal will drop very slightly due to the overlap.

Cross-talk causes a very slight loss of signal in the adjacent slice. So, exciting slice 1 also excites a little bit of slice 2. Then, when slice2 is excited, a little bit of it has already been excited and slice 2 gives just a little less signal than it should. This has minimal impact on IQ but is a real event. You would notice this signal loss more on T1 weighted imaging because of the short TR. Figure 12.20 depicts three slices. Each slice has an overlap in transmitter B/W frequencies.

The other "cross-talk" happens in spines with steep angles with slices that overlap. This can be more accurately termed "cross-excitation," but everybody calls it cross-talk.

Control of Cross-talk

There are ways to combat slice cross-talk. You can use a **gap** to separate slices a little bit or **interleave** the slices. Gap is easy, it is a percentage of the slice thickness that is not scanned in between slices (Figure 12.21).

The other way is to "interleave" the slices. You can tell the scanner to acquire every other slice, then fill in the missing ones. Figure 12.22 shows slices 1, 3, and 5 acquired first, then 2 and 4 next. This interleaving is actually a 100% gap as a full slice is skipped in order to eliminate cross-talk, then the missing pieces are filled in.

You can also add a gap to an interleaved acquisition slice order, making it a 100% plus gap. Cross-talk is rarely if ever seen or noticed these days. Advancements in RF transmitters and RF filters have made the RF pulse almost square.

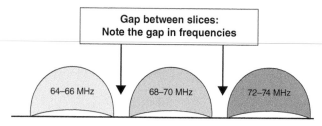

Figure 12.21 The fix for "cross-talk" is to shift the slices away from each other or place a gap between them. There will be a small percentage of tissue that is not imaged.

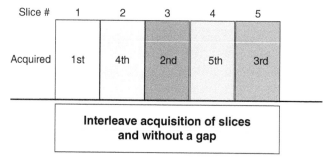

Figure 12.22 An alternative fix for cross-talk is to interleave the slice acquisition order. Basically you "skip" every other slice, then go back and fill in the skipped slices. Example: 1, 3, 5, 7, 9, 2, 4, 6, 8. A combination of a gap and interleaved slices is also not unheard of.

Cross-excitation

You have seen this many times. We all call it cross-talk, but I prefer to describe it as **cross-excitation.** It occurs when slices cross each other with little time for T1 relaxation of the common tissue (Figures 12.23–12.25).

This artifact can be reduced by altering the angle of the lower stack for less overlap or making one larger stack to cover both disc spaces. Both of these will not follow the rule of "angling to the disc." The correct way is to scan the lower stack (slices 7–9) separately to have no cross-excitation (Figures 12.26 and 12.27).

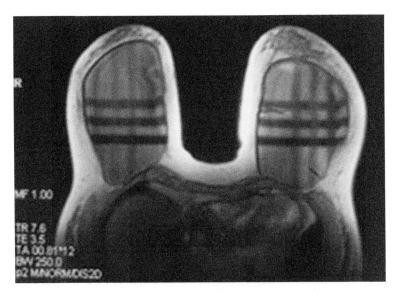

Figure 12.23 Cross-excitation artifact: Dark bands on scouts in breast implants.

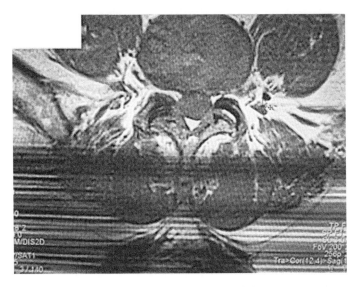

Figure 12.24 Cross-excitation: Overlapping of slices posterior to the spine.

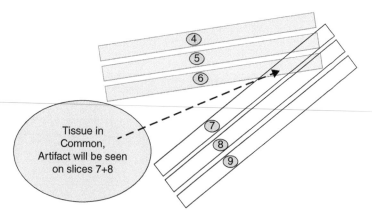

Tissue in Common, Artifact will be seen on slices 7+8

Figure 12.25 Schematic showing the overlapping of slices causing the artifact in Figure 12.24.

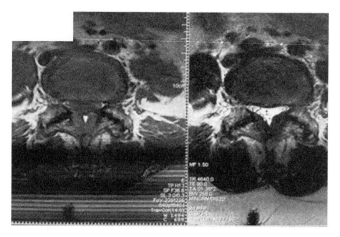

Figure 12.26 Same slices and patient. Cross-excitation in T1s on the left, seen to a much lesser extent on T2s on the right. **The reason is the long TR.** It gives tissues much more time to T1 relax.

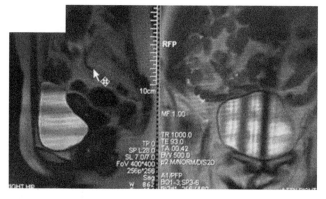

Figure 12.27 Urinary bladder with cross-excitation.

Gradient Warp or Distortion

The gradient's job is to change the magnetic field during scanning. It does this very well, but only over a limited distance. The distance a gradient is effective for is not infinite. This artifact is seen on **large FOVs**.

We assume gradients are linear, which they are, but they are only **linear** over a certain distance. They get less linear (less straight) at the edges of the FOV and actually start to return to zero (circled in Figure 12.28).

The artifact appears as a black hole/distortion with the edges of the image elongating or "warping," hence gradient warp (Figures 12.29 and 12.30).

Metal Artifacts

We have all seen metal effects. Metal changes the magnetic field homogeneity. The field actually gets a little stronger, so it changes the PF of the protons. They spin faster. Let's say you are scanning on a 1.5 T. The RF is 63 MHz. Protons at

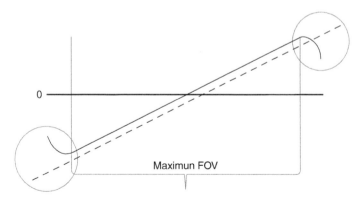

Figure 12.28 The dashed line is the desired FOV. The solid line represents the actual shape of the gradient field. Imaging beyond the maximum FOV is where the gradient field becomes less **linear** and causes warping/distortion of the image. The gradient field is actually starting to fall off and go back to zero (circled).

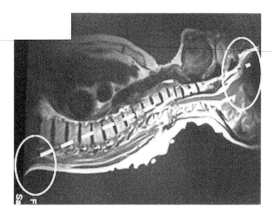

Figure 12.29 Imaging past the linear portion of the gradient results in warp (circled).

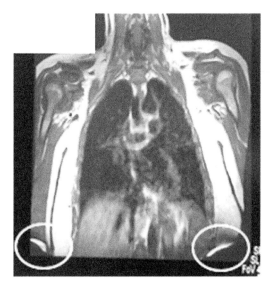

Figure 12.30 Another example of gradient warp (circled).

63 MHz respond, but those near the metal are spinning at say 68 MHz. They do not respond or flip so give no signal. That area is seen as a black/white hole (Figure 12.31). It is a very bad susceptibility artifact and may render some sequences unreadable. As you already know, GRE sequences are the most sensitive to metal.

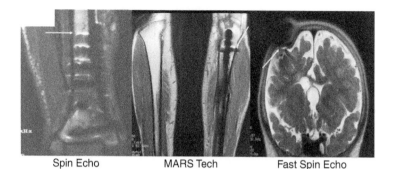

| Spin Echo | MARS Tech | Fast Spin Echo |

Figure 12.31 Metal artifact on scanning with three different sequences: SE, MARS, and FSE. Note lessening of artifact in the middle image scanned with MARS. Also note white "domes" (arrows) at the edges of the artifact. These are typical of metal artifact and are seen in the frequency direction.

Workarounds for Metal Artifact:

- Avoid GREs and fat-sats. Run a STIR instead of a T2 fat-sat.
- Use a "MARS" technique. MARS is a generic technique possible on all sequences and scanners. MARS is a combination of parameter changes to lessen the effects of metal. Those parameters are:
  - Increase the ETL.
  - Widen the receiver B/W.
  - Use the shortest TE possible to decrease the amount of de-phasing. You have to be cognizant not to lower the TE too much on T2s.
  - Use the smallest FOV possible.

Corduroy Artifact

Figure 12.32 shows "corduroy" artifact. It comes from a data point or two which is corrupt in k-space. It can be seen any direction, and on single or multiple slices. Causes include:

- Electromagnetic spikes from gradients or **light bulbs.**
- Electronic equipment in the scan room.

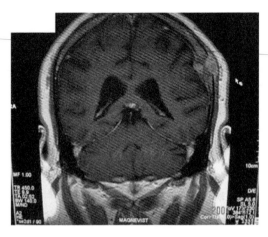

Figure 12.32 Corduroy artifact. This comes from a data point or two which is corrupt in *k*-space. It can be seen any direction, and on single or multiple slices. Causes vary:

- Fluctuating AC power.
- Static electricity in the equipment room from low humidity.

There is really no option but to run the sequence again. If artifact continues, it is a service call.

Annifact

Annifact (Figure 12.33) is often seen on spine exams from signal **from outside the FOV.** It is not phase wrap causing the artifact. **There is too much/too many coil(s) turned on for the FOV (SP2 is the likely cause). SP3–5 are OK.** If you have a 32 FOV and have turned on 48 worth of coil that extra coil will receive signal and that signal has to go somewhere.

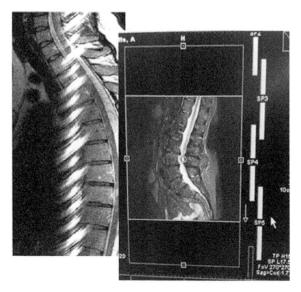

Figure 12.33 Annifact.

Moiré Fringe Artifact or Zebra Artifact

Look at Figure 12.34. Here, in the abdomen, **moiré fringe artifact** comes from a combination of aliasing artifacts and magnetic field inhomogeneities. It is an interference pattern of superimposed images with different phases where the right side wraps in on the left, and the left wraps in on the right, cancelling each other out.

Moiré fringe or zebra artifact is typically seen on steady state-GREs, and large and off-center FOVs.

The main artifact control for this type of artifact is keeping the TR as short as possible. A TR of 4 ms or less is ideal. Multiple things can affect the TR: Flip angle, receiver B/W, phase and frequency matrix, fat-sat, and FOV.

- Manual shim when possible, and use two small shims if possible. Some systems now have this feature.
- Auto pre-scan also helps as these sequences love to drift off from the center frequency.

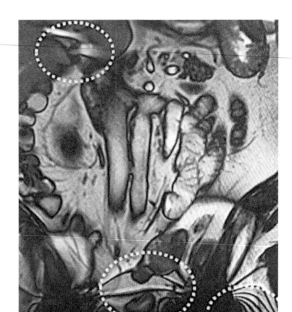

Figure 12.34 Moiré fringe or zebra artifact.

■ The artifact is worse with fat-sat because the TR gets longer and SNR also drops.

Magnetic Susceptibility Artifact

Magnetic susceptibility is a tissue's ability to be magnetized. Is it susceptible to a magnet or does it fight it like air? Most human tissue is susceptible, air is not. When different tissues of varying susceptibilities meet, this artifact occurs. (Slice location in Figure 12.35 is just above the sphenoid sinus, same slice, same patient.)

Susceptibility artifacts are worse on GREs because there is no 180° RF pulse(s). Figure 12.36 shows multiple weightings with different degrees of artifact severity.

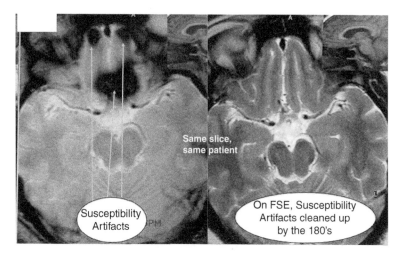

Figure 12.35 Magnetic susceptibility from air in the paranasal sinuses. The multiple 180°s in a TSE help to correct or lessen this artifact.

(A)   (B)   (C)   (D)   (E)

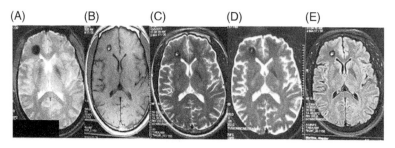

Figure 12.36 Right frontal hemorrhage on all weightings: A, GRE; B, T1 FSE; C, T2 FSE; D, B_0-DWI; E, T2 FLAIR.

Reminder: 180°s clean up for the Big Three by putting the protons into phase at TE. De-phased protons = decreased signal.

Dielectric Effect or Standing Wave

This is a somewhat unique/rare artifact. It is theoretically possible at all fields, however it is mostly seen at 3 T. This artifact has its roots in inhomogeneities of the B_1 or RF field in the patient.

Let's pull apart the name: "Di," meaning two, in combination with "electric," equals "two-electrics" or two electric fields. Looking at the image (Figure 12.37), the signal loss comes from the two electric fields canceling each other out. That is quite simple, right? But why two fields?

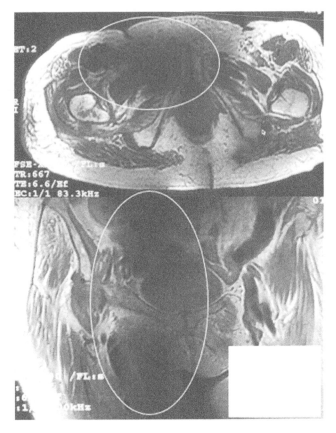

Figure 12.37 Dielectric effect" (circled) in the same patient in two different planes. Both images scanned at 3 T.

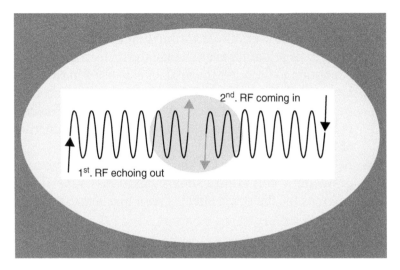

Figure 12.38 A simplified depiction of the dielectric effect. The large oval represents the slice. The first RF has already been applied and is echoing out when the second RF is applied and is entering the slice. The circle where they meet is the "shading" caused by the two RFs cancelling each other out. **Note the arrows are going in different directions.**

A physicist once explained it to me this way: Due to the wavelength of the RF at 3 T when it goes into the human body (with large FOVs) it is more likely that the RF will "echo back out." While **one RF** is echoing out, **another RF** pulse is coming in (Figure 12.38). Here they cause a cancelling out effect, signal loss, or what is often described as "shading."

"Standing wave" is another way to describe the dielectric effect. Two RF waves are present **simultaneously or "standing", so "standing wave."**

There are a few things to know about the dielectric effect:

- RF likes to go into round things. You tend to see the dielectric effect artifact in very large or very thin patients.
- Ascites and amniotic fluid seem to make it even more likely (something to do with the chemical make-up of the fluids).

- A large FOV tends to increase the dielectric effect.
- Note in your everyday scanning that small FOV IACs or pituitaries seldom if ever display the dielectric effect.
- An option to decrease the artifact is to use a hard-to-find item called dielectric pads. Dielectric pads are placed between the patient and the coil. They have a gel-like solution of manganese chloride which increases the conductivity of RF into the patient.
- Be careful not to confuse the dielectric effect with a coil problem. A coil failure shows signal loss superficially whereas the dielectric effect is seen inside the image.

Magic Angle Artifact

The "magic angle" artifact is subtle and actually not so rare. It is an interesting artifact that you probably see often but do not notice. For magic angle artifact to happen, two specific conditions need to be present:

- *A tendon/ligament orientated at 55° to B_0.*
- *A short TE*. Magic angle artifact is only seen on T1 and PD weighted sequences.

This artifact is not a "call-back" kind of thing. There is not much you can do to eliminate the artifact. You can take some steps to keep the tendon off 55° with positioning if you like. Do not re-invent the wheel by positioning the patient differently or taking out a protractor.

As for the TE, TEs above 35–40 ms tend to minimize the artifact. A note on the TEs often used in PDs in a musculoskeletal (MSK) exam: The TEs are now considered "hybrids" (not quite the traditional PD but not quite a T2. This is due to an effective TE of 35 ms or more and an ETL of 5–8. Magic angle artifact is not seen on T2s. **Magic angle artifact is often seen on fat-sat images.**

Magic angle appears as a bright signal, usually seen in either the supraspinatus tendon or the patellar tendon at their insertions (Figures 12.39 and 12.40). The artifact is not limited to just those

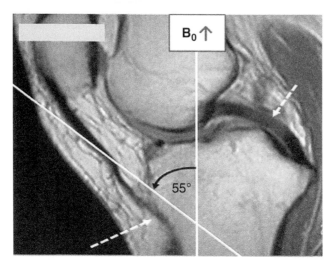

Figure 12.39 The patellar tendon at 55° to the main magnetic field (MMF) on the T1 weighted image. Note the higher than expected signal in the patellar tendon as well as the posterior cruciate ligament (arrows).

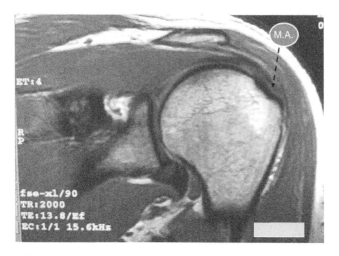

Figure 12.40 The dashed arrow points to the magic angle artifact (M.A.) in the supraspinatus tendon on this PD weighted oblique coronal image of the shoulder. This magic angle artifact is not often seen or talked about now with the use of "hybrid" PD weighted sequences in musculoskeletal (MSK) protocols.

tendons, however. Any ligament or tendon with a lot of collagen at 55° (54.7° to be exact) can demonstrate the artifact. The artifact is known to radiologists, who just "read through" it. They will see bright signal in the tendon on a T1 or PD. If it goes away on the T2s it is magic angle. If it persists, it is pathology.

Teaching Moment: Bright fluid on T1? The things that are bright on a T1 are fat, gadolinium, and proteins. If the bright area were true pathology, it would be bright on a T2 also. Magic angle goes away because of the TE. Pathology (fluid) is bright on T2 weighted images. The body reacts to an insult by forcing fluids to the area.

Why do we get magic angle artifact? In the literature, you will see the terms **"dipole coupling" or "dipole vector coupling."** What these mean is that trace amounts of water align along "ordered collagen" (ligaments or tendons) and under specific conditions such as TEs below 35 ms and the structure being at 55° to the main magnetic field. These conditions can and will give you bright water signal on a T1. This **"coupling"** or adding up of water's NMV actually shortens the T2 time of water, which produces signal at short TEs. Water is never bright on a T1 unless it is mixed with something. At longer TEs, 35 ms and higher, this "coupling" effect goes away. Remember: Artifacts are false or incorrect information seen in an image.

A question I have been asked is: How do you know the tendon is at 55° to the main magnetic field? You will not know until you get some images. At that point do you start measuring angles or repositioning the patient? **No.** Everybody's anatomy is a bit different and you will only occasionally see magic angle artifact. As mentioned previously, this is a subtle artifact and you will not be calling the patient back because of it. Just know that it exists and you will occasionally see it.

Notes

13

Gradients

Chapter at a Glance

Physical Gradients
   The Cartesian Coordinate System
   Physical Gradients: How They Work
Logical Gradients
   Spatial Encoding: Slice Selection
   Spatial Encoding: Phase Encoding
   Spatial Encoding: Frequency Encoding

The subject of gradients is one of the most feared and avoided topics for most MR Technologists. It is also one of the most difficult to understand.

How many patients have asked you: "What makes all that noise?"? Your stock answer is: "Those are 'the gradients'." Now, what if they ask: "What is a gradient?"? Your answer is: "It's a hill, a magnetic hill to be precise." The noise results from the X, Y, and Z gradients being turned on and off very rapidly with a very large amount of electricity. You get a bang when they are turned on, and one when they are turned off. Three gradients turned on

MRI Physics: Tech to Tech Explanations, First Edition. Stephen J. Powers.
© 2021 John Wiley & Sons Ltd. Published 2021 by John Wiley & Sons Ltd.

and off rapidly equals six loud bangs in a time span of usually less than 4 s for a T2, and less than three quarters of a second for T1.

The "magnetic hills" come from the "physical X, Y, Z gradients" being turned on and off. The X, Y, and Z gradients physically exist inside the bore. They are physical things that you can touch. The slice, phase, and frequency encodings that I have talked about so often so far are called the "logical gradients." The logical gradients you need to think about. The logical aspect is which physical gradient is doing which job: Slice, phase, or frequency encoding.

- *Physical Gradients:* The X, Y, Z. These exist in the bore of the scanner and are turned on and off rapidly to perform three different tasks: Slice, phase and frequency encoding.
- *Logical Gradients:* Which of the three is doing which task? Each gradient can do any of the three.

Physical Gradients

As previously stated, a gradient is a hill. One end is "high," the other "low." The three gradients cross or pivot at isocenter. Isocenter is where we ideally do all our imaging.

> **FYI:** Every gradient is used during a pulse sequence. They can all do any of the encoding jobs of slice, phase, and frequency.

The physical gradients are in the bore of the scanner; you can touch them. They live in the "gradient coil," which is buried inside the bore amongst others. The gradient coil holds the actual loops of wire that are the X, Y, and Z gradients. These gradients are turned on and off very rapidly during the pulse sequence to encode slice, phase, or frequency. The other coils inside the bore are the "body coil," which transmits the RF for most imaging exams, and the "shim coils," of which there are two: a "hard shim coil and a "soft or electronic shim." We want a very homogeneous magnetic field. The magnet sitting there alone with no patient in it is very homogeneous. The field engineers make sure of it on install and check it each time the engineer performs preventative maintenance (PM). When you add in a human body, things change. The patient is a big disrupter of magnetic field inhomogeneity. The shim coils can adjust the field to make it more uniform.

The Cartesian Coordinate System

The next concept to understand in gradients is the **Cartesian coordinate system**. The three cardinal directions are X, Y, and Z, where X is right/left (R/L) and Y is up/down (in MRI that is anterior/posterior – A/P). There is also a third direction, Z. Remember how we did this in school, on graph paper? From zero, we moved our pencil -2X and +3Y. These dimensions are referred to as an "axis," that is, the X, Y, and Z axis. The X and Y directions are the same ones you learned in school; the third dimension, Z, runs the length of the bore or superior/inferior (S/I). In Figure 13.1 you can see my left hand/fingers as an example. Picture yourself sitting scanning and looking up the bore. Your thumb is pointing to your nose. My former students are shaking their heads and saying "Here we go."

Qualities a Gradient Needs: There are three essential qualities gradients must have: Linearity, constancy, and reproducibility.

- *Linearity* means it is straight.
- *Constancy* means its strength does not waver during application.
- *Reproducibility* means it is the same every TR.

Linearity is a key aspect: If a gradient is non-linear, images look warped. See the section in Chapter 12 on "Gradient Warp or Distortion."

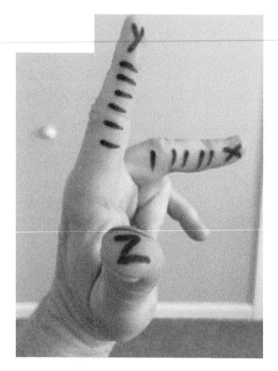

Figure 13.1 A photo of my **left** hand with the X, Y, and Z physical gradient directions shown. X = R/L; Y = A/P; Z = S/I.

Physical Gradients: How They Work

When a gradient is applied, **it temporarily alters the main magnetic field by adding to one end or side while subtracting from the other end or side.**

The example in Figure 13.2 is just one direction of field change. Remember, there are three of them. The other two in the patient (bore) are L/R from the X, and A/P from the Y.

You may have noticed that the sound changes due to different TR/TE/TI combinations and whether the sequence is very "gradient intense" or more "RF intense." As an example, listen to the sound from a DWI being gradient intense vs. a conventional or fast spin echo. Over time, you will be able to tell what sequence is running without even looking at the control screen.

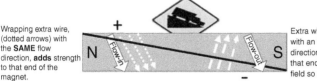

Wrapping extra wire, (dotted arrows) with the **SAME** flow direction, **adds** strength to that end of the magnet.

Extra wire (dashed arrows) with an **OPPOSED flow** direction **subtracts** from that end main magnetic field so is weaker.

Here a stronger field is created on the left, where current adds to magnet strength and weaker to the right where the current opposes the flow and weakens the main mag. field.

Figure 13.2 A magnet's strength comes from the amount of current flowing in the wires. More wire with current equals a stronger magnet. When simultaneously energized, the extra magnetic field generated to the left (north) adds to the main magnetic field (MMF) while the extra wire on the right (south) with opposing current flow subtracts from the MMF. A magnetic field gradient is produced.

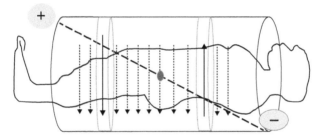

Figure 13.3 Z gradient, side view. The patient is silhouetted in the bore. The dot represents isocenter. Current flow in the main magnet is the dotted arrows. Solid arrows depict direction of flow in the Z gradients. The left end adds to the magnetic field while flow at the right end opposes the flow in the main magnetic field, subtracting from the main field.

Physical Gradient "Z"

Figure 13.3 is a representation of the effects of turning on the "Z" gradient. The Z gradient is used for axial slices. The patient is head first, supine. Turning on the Z gradient adds to the foot end and subtracts from the head end. Tissue by the knees, seeing a stronger magnetic field, temporarily speeds up (higher PF), while the head end sees a lower magnetic field. They then slow (a lower PF) due to the weaker magnetic field. This is spatial encoding for axials. In a PSD for axial slices, the Z gradient is applied during RF excitation. Please note that the gradient strength changes with the amount of electricity flowing. Also know that the Z gradient, like all gradients, can be reversed. This example showed the head end being the weak end, and the foot end the strong end. The head end can be strong while the foot end is weak. They are not always in the same direction. The dot at about the patient navel represents "isocenter." If you look back at Figure 13.1, Z is my thumb, the long axis of the bore.

Again, this a **short and temporary** altering of the main magnetic field in the S/I, longitudinal, or Z axis.

Physical Gradient "X"

I described the Z gradient first because it is the easiest to understand. The other two are the same principle of adding and subtracting from the main magnetic field, but in different directions. The X gradient would be used for slice encoding the field R/L for sagittals (Figures 13.4 and 13.5). The physical shape of both the X and Y gradients is not a "donut" shape like the Z, but a curved rectangle. It is able to add/subtract to the main magnetic field from right to left. In Figure 13.1, this is my middle finger.

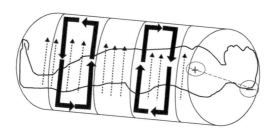

Figure 13.4 X gradient, side view. There are identical coils on opposite sides of the bore. Current flow in the main magnet is in the direction of the dotted arrows. Solid arrows show the direction of flow in the X gradients. The near side **adds to** the magnetic field (say, the patient's **left**) while flow on the opposite side of the bore opposes or **subtracts from** the main magnetic field on the patient's **right** side. At isocenter the magnetic field strength is not affected. This is what happens. Away from isocenter the precessional frequency (PF) changes from right to left for slice selection.

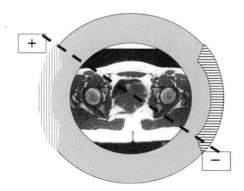

Figure 13.5 X gradient, sagittals. You are looking up the bore scanning sagittals through the pelvis. The patient is head first and supine. The right hip is on the high or strong side of the gradient so will have a higher PF compared to the left side which has a lower PF.

Physical Gradient "Y"

The Y gradient is used to slice encode for coronals (Figures 13.6 and 13.7). It can make the **anterior/top** of the magnetic field stronger than the **posterior** side (or vice versa). The Y has the same physical shape as the X gradient; it is on the top and bottom of the bore. In Figure 13.1, this is my index finger.

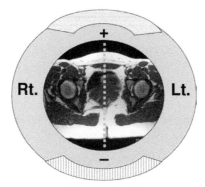

Looking up the Bore

Figure 13.6 Y gradient, coronals. Coils at the top of the main magnetic field (MMF) cause the field to increase, whereas the coils posteriorly subtract from the MMF causing a field gradient to form anteriorly–posteriorly (A/P) for slice selection of coronals.

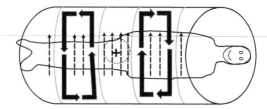

Figure 13.7 Y gradient seen from above. The patient is silhouetted supine in the scanner. There are identical coils on the top and bottom of the bore. Current flow in the main magnet is in the direction of the dashed arrows. Solid arrows depict the direction of flow in the Y gradients. Here, the top adds to the magnetic field anteriorly, while flow on the bottom aspect of the bore opposes the flow in the MMF, thus subtracting from the main field posteriorly.

Logical Gradients

As I said earlier, you need to think (be logical) about these.

As already mentioned, these three gradients do the jobs of slice selection, phase encoding, and frequency encoding. Any one of them can do any of these jobs. I have already covered a portion of this logical gradient idea, that being the slice selective portion (SSG) of the three cardinal planes: Axial, coronal, and sagittal. That being said, while one gradient is doing SSG, the other two will have to do either phase encoding (PEG) or frequency encoding (FEG).

An easy start here is axials in the abdomen. Again, and as usual, the patient is head first and supine. Off the coronal scout, you position axials to cover the liver. You have made the Z gradient the SSG. The other two, X and Y, will then be the PEG and FEG. If you were to set up coronals, then the Y gradient would be the SSG and the Z and X would be PEG and FEG. In the same way, if you set up sagittals, then X will be SSG, so Z and Y will be PEG and FEG.

The thinking part concerns which gradient performs which function. The SSG is easy; it is the other two that can be daunting. OK, so you have covered the dome of the liver to the bottom of the kidneys with axials. The general rule in MR is to have the phase direction in the short axis of the body so for that, phase is

A/P. The Y gradient picks up this job (PEG), leaving X for FEG. For the most part, we are smaller A/P than L/R.

The reason for having the PEG in the short axis is to save time. If the phase direction is in the short axis, whether it is R/L, A/P, or S/I, you can employ a rectangular FOV to save some time and not worry about wrap too much. You also need to know which phase is as that is the motion direction. **Note here that scanners default to frequency R/L or X direction.** In the brain, for example, when you set up axials, the Z is SSG. This automatically puts frequency in the R/L and phase in the A/P. That is convenient in the abdomen with frequency R/L but in the brain we are "longer" A/P than R/L. In this case, we want phase and frequency to go the other way so we can tell the scanner to change the default direction to: PEG is R/L, and FEG is A/P. Recall, any gradient can do any job.

Some vendors tell you the phase direction, others tell you the frequency direction. Neither is more correct. This is just the way they do it. Motion and wrap are always seen in the phase direction so there are times where you may want to "swap" phase and frequency to make motion go in the other direction and also have consideration for the phase direction, watching out for wrap or aliasing.

Figure 13.8 is an axial in the brain, showing that the brain is longer A/P than it is R/L. If we kept the default R/L frequency, putting phase A/P, we would not be able to save time with a Rec. FOV without wrap.

Some Gradient FYIs:

- All gradients are used during a sequence.
- Each TR, they are always the same strength and duration. PEG is the exception during a 2D.
- During a sequence, each gradient has a specific job: Slice, phase, and frequency encoding.
- These jobs can be thought of as the "logical gradients."
- Any gradient can do any job.

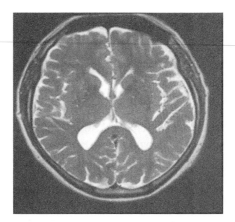

Figure 13.8 The gradient directions on this axial image of the brain were "swapped," changing their directions by 90°. This was done to allow taking advantage of a narrower body part and saving some time. Phase was made R/L instead of A/P. The image is windowed to show the rectangular FOV, which is R/L.

Spatial Encoding: Slice Selection

The next and final concept to be covered under gradients is what is called spatial encoding. It is not really that hard and we have already partially covered a portion of it: Slice selection. That is where I shall start. I shall ask you to re-look at Figure 13.1 from time to time.

Figures 13.9 and 13.10 are FSE PSD with RF pulses and gradient pulses labeled. This "logical" gradient concept can be difficult, but with some thought and practice you can get it. Hopefully, the PSDs will now make more sense than they did earlier in the book.

Let me start out by saying that, in a perfect world or with a perfect magnet of, say, 1.5 T, the entire patient is precessing at 63 MHz. We all know that the patient is the biggest cause of field inhomogeneity so the previous statement cannot be true, but let's just go with a perfect magnet. Gradients are turned on then off to do their job(s). Seldom are two gradients on simultaneously.

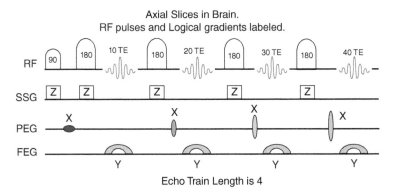

Figure 13.9 An FSE pulse sequence with an ET of 4. The Z gradient is slice select (long axis of the magnet). X is phase, applied between the 90° and 180°. Y is the frequency encoding applied during echo formation.

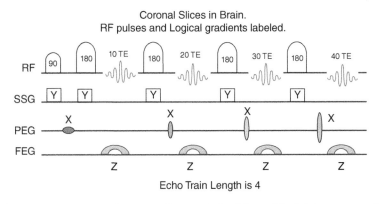

Figure 13.10 Same PSD as in Figure 13.9 with an ET of 4, but coronal slices. The Y gradient is slice select (A/P). X is phase, applied between the 90° and 180°. Z is the frequency encoding applied during echo formation.

In Figure 13.10, turning on the SSG (Z) alters the field S/I. Recall that the patient is assumed to be head first and supine in the scanner unless otherwise stated. Five axial slices are prescribed in the brain as shown in Figure 13.11. Tissues at the strong end temporarily speed up (an increase in PF) and the top slice goes to 65 MHz; at the low end, they slow down (lowered PF) to 61 MHz. The middle slice is at 63 MHz. You really do not know which way the field is being changed, S/I or I/S; it does not matter. The scanner knows, but we do not. During "pre-scan" the scanner tunes to the RF of the center slice (63 MHz) of your stack of slices and can then calculate out the RF frequencies above or below the center slice.

At the start of the sequence, a 90° and 180° RF pulse of 65 MHz is applied during the SSG that matches the top slice's PF and excites that slice only. The others do not respond as they are precessing at less than 65 Mhz. They are not at that PF (65 MHz) due to their location along the SSG. Their turn will come. Phase encoding happens between the 90° and 180°s, frequency encoding at the TE.

The above is an example of the center frequencies at 61–65 MHz for the slices is extremely oversimplified for ease in explanation and understanding. Remember that each slice is a transmitted range of precessional frequencies (+/-).

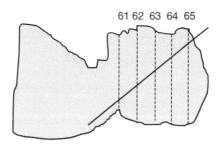

61 62 63 64 65

5 Slices along the SSG: Dotted lines

Figure 13.11 SSG is applied, the top slice is excited with a 90° RF at 65 MHz, phase encoded, SSG, 180° RF at 65 MHz, then frequency encoded at TE. The process is repeated for the next slice down: SSG A 90° at 64 MHz, phase encoded, SSG, 180'd at 64 MHz, frequency encoded at TE.

Spatial Encoding: Phase Encoding

The phase encoding of the future echo happens between the 90° and 180° RF pulses. PEG is applied orthogonal or at 90° to the slice. The Phase Encoding Gradient is very slightly altered each TR to make each echo just slightly out of phase with or out of sync with the next echo. Its duration of application is fixed; the amplitude or strength is altered. Another way to think of phase is that it makes the echoes not synchronized. If everybody is doing the same thing at the exact same time, they are said to be in phase or in sync. Each echo acquired at TE is a slightly different phase from the previous one. This is done by the PEG. It is the same echo and same slice; it just has a very slightly different phase. This difference is vital to put each echo into a different line of k-space (Figure 13.12).

In a conventional SE sequence, the PEG is changed in amplitude each TR. In the case of an FSE sequence, the PEG

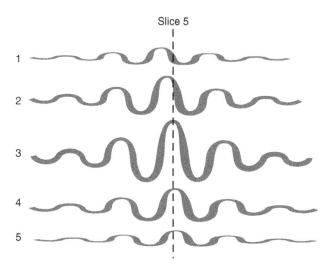

Figure 13.12 Five echoes, same frequency. Five different phases from five different strengths of the PEG. The dotted line is placed to show that the five echoes cross at a different point and are **out of phase** with each other.

is slightly altered for each echo in the echo train. There are as many phase gradient applications as you have number of phase steps in your scan matrix: 256 × 192 has 192 phase applications, 256 × 128 has 128 phase applications.

Should the PEG not be altered for each echo, all the echoes would be exactly the same and go into the same line of k-space.

Any given sequence runs until all the phase lines in k-space are filled. At that point, when k-space is filled, the array processor takes the data and processes it into the images. When you look at a line diagram of a PSD, you will notice that the PEG is shown as in Figure 13.13, either square or parabolic. This represents that the gradient varied in amplitude. Note that on a 3D sequence, the SSG is also shown like this. This denotes the "locs" (locations) or partitions.

Above the line is a positive gradient, below is negative. What is seldom mentioned is that there is a TR when no PEG is turned on. A zero gradient is still different from the -1 before it and the +1 after it. A 256-phase matrix will have 128+ applications, a 0, then 127- applications. This equals 256 phases.

Phase Encoding: Part 2

I have alluded that there are positive (+) and negative (-) phase steps and that also there is a "zero" phase step, where no phase gradient is applied. That means that no phase is imparted into

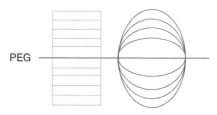

Slice 5 has 5 phase encodings

Figure 13.13 The five PEGs vary in strength from high negative applications below the line to high positive above the line. Note that the length of time that the PEG is applied is constant. Only the amplitude varies.

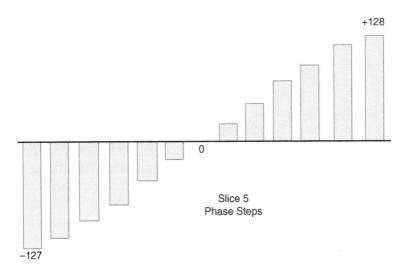

Figure 13.14 A truncated PEG playout of steps: –127 to 0, and then out to phase step +128. High negative amplitude phase steps put the echo in the outer lines on one side of the *k*-space, the lower PEGs place the echoes into the center lines, and high positive phase steps fill out the remaining lines. High amplitude phase steps equal low amplitude echoes, and vice versa.

that echo. That is right, there is no phase – it is still a different phase when compared to the one before and the one after it.

The sequence starts out with the negative phase steps, meaning that the highest negative phase steps are applied first, moving through 0 and out through the positive. There is always a zero phase step. Example: -127, -126, -125, . . . 0, +1, +2, +3, +4, +5 . . . +126, +127, +128. This example of -127 to 0 and +128 equals 256 phase steps (Figure 13.14).

Spatial Encoding: Frequency Encoding

Frequency encoding is the last of the three dimensions: Slice first, phase second, and frequency third. It is also applied at 90° or orthogonal to both the PEG and SSG. The FEG is applied during the TE. The frequency of the signals being acquired is dependent on their location within the FOV. If that last sentence does not make any sense to you, you are not alone.

You might be saying, "Wait, you're changing the frequency?" Yes, pretty much. Remember you already know the slice, and the phase. Frequency is the third coordinate needed to place the exact source of the signal.

In high school you learned at least two coordinates, X and Y. In MR, we have three: X, Y, and Z (see Figure 13.1). We know what slice location the echo is coming from, along the Z gradient in this case. We did the phase encoding with the X gradient, and finally frequency encoding comes from the Y. We have the three points to "triangulate" a signal's location. So, with the final piece of the equation, the frequency encoding, we know that in Figure 13.11 a signal came from slice 5 in the Z axis, -6X in phase, and +4Y in frequency. The next echo would be slice 5, -5X, and +4 frequency. We know where the echo originated.

When the SSG is applied, it sets the PF of your slices. Every time it is applied in a sequence; its strength is the same. The 90° RF excites a slice, let's say slice 5. So, we know which k-space the eventual echo will go into. We have one of the three coordinates needed for echo location. The PEG is applied after the 90°. It puts a "phase" into the transverse NMV. Let's just say it is a high positive step. That phase is used to know in which line, up or down, the echo will be placed. In Figure 13.15 this is line 1. We now have two out of three coordinates. During the TE, the FEG is turned on orthogonal to the phase direction. It changes the frequencies across the slice. Yes, it changes the frequencies. That is OK because we know the slice and the phase line. This is what I could not wrap my head around when I was learning spatial encoding. Changing the frequencies? No, you can't do that! But yes, we can.

The FEG gives us the third coordinate we need to locate the echo in the patient. If you think about it, why can't we just frequency encode once and be done with it? We can't. We need to have a combination of phase and frequency encodings in orthogonal planes to collect all the spatial information. Having only one frequency reading would make the data ambiguous and probably corrupt. IQ would suffer.

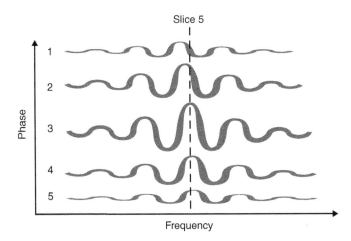

Figure 13.15 A representation of the *k*-space for slice 5. In it we have a phase matrix of 5. From TR #1, a 90° RF pulse causes a free induction decay (FID) that will eventually become the echo and go into *k*-space #5, but where? The first PEG labels it into line #1, and the FEG gives us the frequencies across the slice. TR #2 applies another 90° RF pulse that gives an FID. PEG #2 is applied a little less strongly this time than the first one and that puts it in line 2, a bit closer to the center lines. FEG #2 maps the frequencies across the slice. TR #3 repeats the same steps, as do TRs 4 and 5. Re-look at the echoes in Figure 13.14, same slice, same frequency, but different phases.

Notes

14

MRI Math

Chapter at a Glance

The Larmor Equation: $W_0 = \gamma B_0$
Acquisitions or Nex or NSA
Scan Time Equations
Pixel Size and Voxel Volume
    Resolution: Pixel Size
    Voxel Volume
How to Convert Hz per Pixel to MHz
In and Out of Phase TEs
Dixon Method or Technique
SNR and the 3D Sequence

Figuring out math equations is not something we do on a routine basis while scanning, but you should have a basic understanding of it. This is basic knowledge you will need when you sit for the MR Advanced Registry.

MRI Physics: Tech to Tech Explanations, First Edition. Stephen J. Powers.
© 2021 John Wiley & Sons Ltd. Published 2021 by John Wiley & Sons Ltd.

The Larmor Equation: $W_0 = \gamma B_0$

The most important number you need to know in MRI is the gyromagnetic ratio of hydrogen. It is 42.57 MHz at 1 T. **It is a constant, which means it never, ever, changes.** It is used in the Larmor equation. Some texts round this number up to 42.60. This number is the precessional frequency (PF) of hydrogen at 1 T. The Larmor equation is:

$$\text{PF or } W_0 = \text{gyromagnetic ratio} \times \text{field strength}$$

Examples:

- At 0.5 T: $42.57 \times 0.5 = 21.28$ MHz.
- At 0.7 T: $42.57 \times 0.7 = 29.79$ MHz.
- At 1.5 T: $42.57 \times 1.5 = 63.87$ MHz.
- At 3 T: $42.57 \times 3 = 127.71$ MHz.

Acquisitions or Nex or NSA

SNR increases with the square root of the number of nex. What is a nex or average? A nex or number of signals averaged (NSA) is how many times you fill the k-space with concurrent TRs. At 1 nex each line is filled once, at 2 nex it is filled twice, etc.

You might say "I doubled my nex (from 1 to 2) and my scan time doubled but not my SNR. Why?" As stated in Chapter 11, signal is thought to be a "constant," meaning we generate a certain amount of signal each acquisition while noise is at a non-constant level in the background of the system. Noise may be lower on one acquisition, and higher on the next, and maybe even higher still on a third. If you average out the SNR of all the nex, it comes out to the square root of the number of nex (Figure 14.1). As you can see, increasing the nex is an inefficient way to gain SNR.

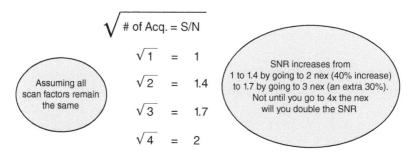

Figure 14.1 Signal to noise changes with the square root of the number of acquisitions.

Scan Time Equations

A lot of people stress about this topic. **First, get the basic Spin Echo scan time formula down.** After that, there are only two others: FSE and 3D. The 2D sequential equation is the same as the 3D, so there are only three equations to learn.

The Basic Scan Time Formula:

TR × number of phase steps × nex = scan time in ms

That math gives a big number, which is the scan time in ms. Now divide that big number of ms by 60,000. **What is that 60,000?** It is the number of ms in 1 min; 1 s is 1000 ms. This step is needed to convert milliseconds into minutes. Now you have a scan time in minutes, something like 3.65 min or 4.7 min. Now keep the minutes (3:), and multiple the .65 by 60, this equals the seconds. The final answer for a scan time of 3.65 min is 3:39.

  Example for a conventional 2D SE sequence:

- 500 ms TR × 192 phase steps × 2 nex = 192,000 ms.
- 192,000 ÷ 60,000 = 3.2 min.
- 3.2 min = 3 min and 2/10ths of a min.

▪ 0.2 × 60 s = 12 s.
▪ The answer is a 3:12 s scan time.

Example for a fast (turbo) SE sequence: FSE has an echo train so that needs to be added to the 2D SE equation.

▪ TR × phase × nex = scan time in ms, then divide by the ETL.
▪ Then divide again by 60,000 = scan time in ms.
▪ 5000 × 192 × 2 = 1,920,000 ms.
▪ 1,920,000 ÷ 7 =274,285 ms.
▪ 274,285 ÷ 60,000 = 4.57 min.
▪ 60 sec × 0.57 = 34 s.
▪ Answer: 4.57 min = 4:34 min.

Convert tenths into seconds. You will need to practice!

3D sequence or 2D sequential scan time formula: Use the basic scan time formula but you need to **factor in the number of partitions or Locs** (locations).

Example for a conventional 3D sequence:

▪ TR × phase × nex × **partitions** (or Locs) = scan time.
▪ 36 × 192 × 1 × **64** = 442,368 ms.
▪ 442,368 ÷ 60,000 = 7.37 min.
▪ 60 s × 0.37 = 22 s.
▪ Answer: 7:22 (7 min and 22 s of scan time).

How about a 2D sequential? **Sequential** is the key word here. A 2D TOF MRA of the carotids is a sequential sequence so use the 3D equation:

▪ TR × phase × nex x number of slices = scan time in ms.
▪ Yes, **it is exactly the same as the 3D.**
▪ 45 × 224 × 1 × 75 = 756,000 ms.
▪ 756,000 ÷ 60,000 = 12.6 min.
▪ 60 × 0.6 = 36 s.
▪ Answer: 12:36 min.

What about an inversion recovery sequence? **If you are asked for an IR sequence, do not use the TI. It is not in the basic scan time formula.** If you are studying for the registry, I strongly suggest that you practice these different formulas. The scanner figures it out for you so do the math yourself and see if it matches the scanner's math. The same thing applies with pixel/voxel size and voxel volume in the next section. When practicing with scan times on the scanner, remove Oversampling, Partial Phase FOV and all Parallel Imaging factors or you scan time math will be way off.

Pixel Size and Voxel Volume

Resolution: Pixel Size

To figure out the pixel size, you apply (divide) the FOV by the scan matrix. So:

$$FOV \div matrix = pixel\ size$$

This math will give you pixel dimensions in width and height.

Example:

- An FOV of 250 or 25, and a matrix of 256×256 (256^2)
- $250 \div 256 = 0.97$ mm in each direction, 0.97×0.97 mm. This is a square or **isotropic** pixel.

What about a not square matrix?

- A 250 FOV and a 192×256 matrix:
- $250 \div 192 = 1.3$ mm
- $250 \div 256 = 0.97$ mm
- The pixel size is 1.3×0.97 mm. This is an **anisotropic** pixel.

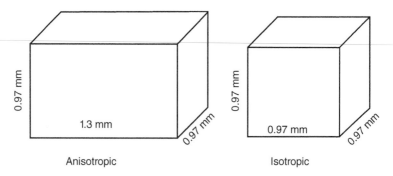

Figure 14.2 The difference between isotropic and anisotropic voxels.

Newer scanners calculate pixel size for you, but I still suggest you practice this math.

Voxel Volume

A voxel is a pixel with a slice thickness, the third dimension. To find a voxel's volume, multiply height by width by thickness. Here is that math for an **isotropic** 0.97 mm voxel (Figure 14.2):

$$0.97 \times 0.97 \times 0.97 = a\ 0.91\,\text{mm}^3 \text{ voxel volume}$$

An anisotropic voxel:

$$1.3 \times 0.97 \times 0.97 = 1.22\,\text{mm}^3 \text{ voxel volume.}$$

Isotropic voxels are ideal for 3D for reformatting.

How to Convert Hz per Pixel to MHz

If you work on two different scanners, like many of us, going back and forth may be difficult if you have Hz per pixel (Hz/Px) and MHz. They are basically the same: Increasing the Hz/Px equals increasing the MHz, you are widening the bandwidth.

If you really want to do the math:

- Take the Hz/Px and multiply by the frequency matrix.
- Then divide by 2.
- Now move the decimal point over to the left three places.
  For example:
- 172 Hz/Px × 256 (frequency matrix) = 44,800.
- 44,800 ÷ 2 = 22,400.
- Move the decimal point over three places = 22.40 kHz.
- 172 × 320 = 55,040.
- 55,040 ÷ 2 = 27,520 = 27.520 kHz.

In and Out of Phase TEs

Where do those numbers come from? The in phase (IP) and out of phase (OOP) TEs that we use vary by field strength. If you have been scanning for a while, you have them memorized as 2.2 ms and 4.4 ms, 6.6 at 1.5 T, and 1.1, 2.2, and 3.3 at 3 T. They are probably saved into the scan protocol, all is well.

In truth, In and Out of Phase TEs are defined by an equation. This equation is seldom if ever mentioned but here it is. The first IP TE is:

$$\frac{1}{3.5\,\mathrm{ppm} \times \mathrm{PF}} \times 1000$$

- First, multiply 3.5 ppm by the PF.
- Second, divide 1 by the above answer.
- Third, multiply by 1000.
- This will equal your first in-phase TE.

What is this 3.5 ppm? In Chapter 12, I explained chemical shift. 3.5 ppm is the numerical difference or shift in PFs between fat and water. This means that for every 1 million (1,000,000) rotations that water does, fat does 3.5 fewer (999,996.5) rotations.

Below is the actual math for a 1.5 T scanner.

Example:

- $1/3.5 \times 63.86 \times 1000 = $ **first IP TE in ms.**
- 3.5×63.68, this equals 223.51.
- Divide 1 by 223.51.
- $1/223.51 = 0.00446$.
- Multiply by 1000 (or just move the decimal point over to the right three places).
- $0.00446 \times 1000 = 4.46$ ms is the first IP TE.

To find the first OOP TE (standard method):

- Take the first IP TE and divide by 2, add the first IP TE.
- $4.46/2 = 2.23$, then add that to the first IP TE.
- $4.46 + 2.23 = 6.69$ ms is the OOP TE.

At 1.5 T we now use the first OOP TE of 2.2–2.3 ms. This is because years ago gradients were not as fast as they are now, so the first OOP TE obtainable was 6.6 ms. A 2.2 ms TE was not possible back then.

A General Rule on OOP TEs: When acquiring a dual echo sequence, as in the adrenals, always acquire the OOP first and the IP second. That is because of a signal loss as the TE gets longer. As a quick reminder: At 1.5 T, the protons are in phase at 0 ms (we cannot image there), de-phase to OOP by 2.2 ms, become IP again at 4.4 ms, OOP at 6.6 ms, and IP again at 8.8 ms. Do you see a pattern developing there?

Dixon Method or Technique

The Dixon technique is a way to get fat-sat-like images at low fields. It is not a true fat-sat, it just provides fat-sat-like images. This is done mathematically by adding or subtracting the echoes. Again, you will not be doing this math while sitting at the console, but I want you to see the basic math done behind the scenes by the scanner.

As a reminder, the Dixon technique evolved because it was not possible to get good fat-sat at magnetic fields of 0.7 T or lower.

The sequence acquires two echoes, an IP and an OOP, then does some math with them to give you four different contrasts: An IP, an OOP, a water only image that shows tissues with a lot of water, and a fat only image that shows high signal from tissues with a lot of fat.

Dixon Math: This is very simplified and displayed so you can have a basic idea on how the "fat only" and "water only" images are produced):

1. IP = (water + fat).
2. OOP = (water − fat).
3. Fat only = IP − OOP = (water + fat) − (water − fat).
4. Water only = IP + OOP = (water + fat) + (water − fat).

SNR and the 3D Sequence

As you already know, a 3D sequence, all factors being the same, has a higher SNR than a 2D sequence. It also has a better resolution owing to its thinner slices or locations.

There are a number of ways to describe the "slices" in a 3D. First, think of a 3D slab as a very big thick slice divided into lots of little slices (Figure 14.3). These little slices are referred to as partitions, locations, Locs, or slices. Now the math.

SNR in a 3D increases with the number of locations or partitions. You may have noticed that the SNR in a 3D goes up as you add slices-or another slab. Scan time goes up at the expense of coverage. The net gain or loss of SNR is the square root of the number of partitions.

As an example: Let's say you have a slab with 36 locations. Here, the SNR of a 3D slab equals the square root ($\sqrt{}$) of 36 which

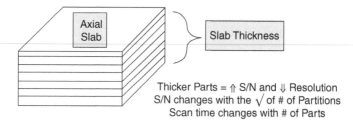

Figure 14.3 Think of a 3D slab as a big, thick slice. That slice is divided into "partitions" or "Locs" by an additional slice select gradient. 3D sequences inherently have higher SNR and resolution compared to a 2D sequence.

comes out to 6. Let's think of "6" as a baseline or 100%. If you need more coverage and increase the number of partitions to 64, the square root of 64 is 8. That is about a 35% **increase** in SNR. Obviously 8 is more than 6. I found the "35%" by doing a simple ratio: 6 is to 100 as 8 is to X.

The number "6" we got from the math does not really mean much until you compare it to the "8" we got from adding partitions to the 3D and re-doing the √ math. That math I just did shows you how the number of slices or partitions in a 3D will affect the SNR of the sequence (not to mention the scan time which has now doubled). The SNR goes up in a 3D with the addition of partitions because you are making the slab thicker. **You can think of the 3D slab and one very thick slice,** which gets "partitioned" by the slice select gradient. Just as in a 2D sequence, when you make the slices thicker, you increase the SNR because you are making the pixels bigger and there are more protons in a thicker slice.

Adding slices to a **sequential 2D** sequence does not increase SNR. It just makes the sequence longer. More slices mean more work (more TRs) (not a longer TR, but more of them) for the scanner, and more work means a longer scan time. Making the slices thicker in a 2D will increase SNR but cost you resolution. Remember, nothing is free in MRI.

Notes

15 Parallel Imaging

Chapter at a Glance

Parallel Imaging: What Is It?

Parallel imaging (PI) lets you image quickly. That's very nice, but how many times have you heard that nothing is free in MRI? Speed comes with a price. **That price is signal.** Speed is great, but be careful, use the speed for good. You cannot use it on everything.

PI fills k-space more efficiently time wise than conventional SE, FSE, or GRE sequences. It allows for fewer phase lines to be filled for a given sequence, thus shortening scan time.

MRI Physics: Tech to Tech Explanations, First Edition. Stephen J. Powers.
© 2021 John Wiley & Sons Ltd. Published 2021 by John Wiley & Sons Ltd.

A Short History of Parallel Imaging: The original PI method from quite a few years ago was called **SMASH: Simultaneous Acquisition of Spatial Harmonics.** Over time, SMASH, with advancements in gradient and coil technology, morphed into something called **SENSE.** Eventually another method was produced called **GRAPPA.**

Both SENSE and GRAPPA do the same thing – shorten scan times – but each has a slightly different way of doing it.

The two basic forms/methods of PI are available from all vendors and they all have their own version of them:

1. *SENSE:* **Sens**itivity Encoding (the old SMASH): GE, ASSET; Siemens, I-Pat/mSense; Philips, SENSE; Hitachi, RAPID; and Toshiba, SPEEDER.
2. *GRAPPA:* **G**ene**r**alized **A**uto-Calibrating **P**artially **P**arallel **A**cquisition: GE, ARC; Siemens, GRAPPA.

When and Where to Use the Speed

- PI is mostly used on the **larger FOVs** like abdomen/pelvis or long bone studies and maybe sagittal thoracic spines, which typically have a higher SNR, vs. small FOVs which do not have an abundance of SNR. I am not a big fan of PI on spine exams due to a small loss of resolution. Consider employing occasionally if you need to lower scan time.
- Small FOV studies (wrist, pituitary, or internal auditory canal (IAC)) are high resolution. The high matrices, thin slices, and small FOV all contribute to a lower SNR anyway so hitting them with PI, which costs more signal loss, is really a no go.
- Another consideration is to use it on those sequences that can handle it (e.g. T1s and PDs). Try to avoid using PI on fat suppressed sequences.

> **Teaching Moment:** Consider fat suppressed sequences to be signal starved. Let's not lose signal twice with PI.

Anytime you do not fill lines of *k*-space, you lose signal. Couple PI with fat-sat and you may find yourself repeating the sequence.

Parallel Imaging: How Does It Work?

SENSE

Lines of *k*-space, are of course, **parallel** to each other, hence the name **parallel imaging**. SENSE uses multiple coil elements and assigns them to image specific lines of *k*-space during the sequence. Multiple coils are imaging multiple lines during scanning instead of them all imaging just one line. This action needs what is called a calibration or coil sensitivity map to be created before the sequence starts (see later).

As an example, the coil has four elements around the anatomy. The scanner assigns:

- Coil 1 to acquire lines 1, 5, 9, 13.
- Coil 2 to acquire lines 2, 6, 10, 14.
- Coil 3 to acquire lines 3, 7, 11, 15.
- Coil 4 to acquire lines 4, 8, 12, 16.

Basically, four lines of phase are filled per TR (kind of like an echo train). Scan time is decreased by a factor of 4, or down to one quarter. More coil elements allow for higher and higher PI factors and more time savings, but again, this speed has a price, and that price is SNR.

In the above SENSE example, scan time is decreased to one quarter, which is a factor of the number of elements in the coil. You can tell the scanner to acquire more or fewer lines to scan faster, or not so fast by asking for fewer lines per TR. The big problem with this method is that if four smaller coils are working to image the entire FOV, you will get wrap. An individual coil just cannot get the entire FOV, so wrap is inevitable.

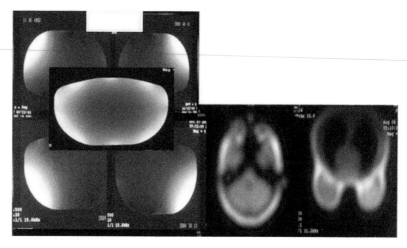

Figure 15.1 Left. Coil sensitivity maps. These provide information to undo the wrap that occurs due to the SENSE method. Bottom right. Brain and breast calibration scans.

This PI filling method (SENSE/ASSET) requires a calibration scan or coil sensitivity map to be performed **prior** to the sequence. The "cal scan" is a low-resolution set of images of a full FOV **that has no wrap** (Figure 15.1). Data from the calibration scan is used to undo the wrap from the individual element data sets. Correction is done after Fourier transform. This is simplified but hopefully you get the general idea.

A Note on the Coil Sensitivity Map/Calibration Scan: If you have to reposition the coil or the patient, a new calibration scan will be needed/should be done. Do not be lazy and pretend you did not move things around. Re-scout, and re-calibrate.

GRAPPA

GRAPPA/ARC are both very similar imaging concepts in that not all the lines of phase are sampled but with one major difference from SENSE. **They do not need calibration scans. They are what is called or do self-calibrating.**

GRAPPA/ARC both fully sample the center lines of k-space, giving good SNR and contrast, but under sample the outer lines to save time (Figure 15.2). The center lines are used as the calibration data. These calibration data are used for filling the outer unsampled lines by something called a "kernel" technique. The kernel technique is like a "spell check" for k-space. It works like this:

If lines A, C, and E are known then B, D, and F can be interpolated.

- Once all the lines of k-space are filled, image processing starts.

- **SNR loss** is a bit less with GRAPPA type imaging (compared to SENSE) as the center lines of k-space are fully sampled and the outer lines are under sampled. Recall, the middle lines contribute the most to overall SNR and image contrast while the edges contribute more to resolution (edge detail).

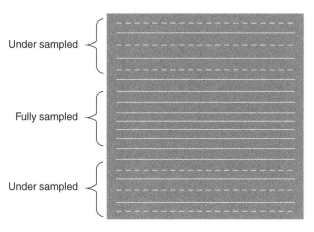

Under sampled

Fully sampled

Under sampled

Figure 15.2 A k-space and how it is filled in the GRAPPA method. The center lines of k-space are fully sampled or filled. Filling all the center lines gives better contrast and SNR as well as for the self-calibrating aspect of GRAPPA. The outer lines are only partially filled with real data, and the "non-filled" lines are filled with what is called a kernel technique **(the dashed lines are not filled).** The GRAPPA method generally works better when getting homogenous sensitivity maps is difficult, as in the chest or abdomen or off-center FOVs.

- The number of lines to **not** fill can be adjusted to shorten scan time. **The more lines not filled will decrease the SNR.** Remember from Chapter 9 on k-space that the center lines of k-space contribute more to contrast and SNR while the outer lines contribute mostly to resolution, but **all** lines contribute to contrast, SNR, and resolution.

Parallel Imaging: Pros and Cons

- Both have slightly lower SNR with decreased scan time.
- The higher the acceleration factor, the lower the SNR.
- The SENSE method is more prone to artifacts/blurring due to a time lapse between the calibration scan and data acquisition. This comes from general patient motion: The coils get moved and the respiratory pattern is different resulting in blurring and mis-registration. If doing manual calibrations, a re-calibration is highly recommended in exams where the cal scan is done early in the study and you are still using those data many sequences later.

What does acceleration factor mean?:

- Basically, it means to go (image) faster.
- An acceleration factor of 2 means half the k-space is sampled; a factor of 3 = one third; 4 = one quarter sampled.

In Figure 15.3 on the right, no acceleration factor has been applied. The left image has an acceleration factor of 2. Note graininess of the image on the left, especially in the cord. Grainy images always mean low SNR. The images are windowed to show lack of SNR.

The effect of high PI factors is shown in Figure 15.4.

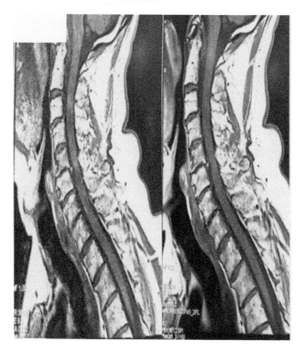

Figure 15.3 Loss of overall SNR. Note graininess of the left image. The right image has good SNR.

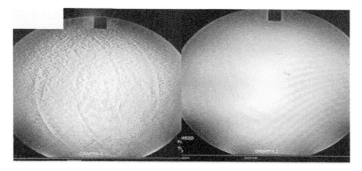

Figure 15.4 Same phantom, parameters, and slice. The right image has PI of 2, the left has 4. Note graininess and ghosting on the left image. It looks like motion, but phantoms do not move. The "zebra" like lines on the right image are from photographing off the scanner's monitor.

Quick PI Review:

- SENSE method: GE, ASSET; Siemens, I-Pat or mSense; Philips, SENSE; Hitachi, RAPID; Toshiba, SPEEDER.
- GRAPPA method: GE, ARC; Siemens, GRAPPA.
- **SENSE** uses a half FOV on the phase direction to save time, so wrap happens. A full FOV cal scan and coil profile data are needed for SENSE to correct the wrap from the half FOV. Corrections are done **after** Fourier transform processing.
- **GRAPPA** samples the center of k-space fully (good SNR and contrast) and partially samples the outer lines. Using a "kernel" method, the outer un-sampled lines are filled in **before** Fourier transform processes the data.

Notes

16 IV Gadolinium

Chapter at a Glance

In this chapter, I shall talk about intravenous (IV) contrast. Cool kids just call it "gad." I am not going to discuss the benefits of one manufacturer's brand over another. That is for the radiologists and Administration to figure out. Neither shall I cover in any great detail nephrogenic systemic fibrosis (NSF), linear or cyclic molecular structure, estimated glomerular filtration rate (eGRF), or anything like that. I shall, however, start out with a short blurb on how renal function is related to NSF/ gadolinium deposition.

MRI Physics: Tech to Tech Explanations, First Edition. Stephen J. Powers.
© 2021 John Wiley & Sons Ltd. Published 2021 by John Wiley & Sons Ltd.

Gadolinium is a toxic "rare earth" metal and is in the periodic table of elements in the lanthanide series. To make gad non-toxic, it is bound to another chemical called a "chelating (pronounced kee-leyt-ing or key-late-ing) agent" DTPA (diethylenetriamine penta acetic acid) or Caldiamide by "Chelation" (pronounced kee-leyt or key-late-shun). What is chelating? Chelation is a way of bonding molecules to a metal ion, that metal being gad. A Ligand or "Ligation" means to "tie to with a ligature".

We know that the kidneys take gad out of the bloodstream by glomerular filtration. If renal function is normal, there is not much of a problem but, if renal function is impaired, the problems can start. When renal function is impaired, and the gad stays in the bloodstream too long, over time the chemical bonds between the chelating agent and gad break down, releasing free gadolinium ions into the body. Gad molecules are too small on their own to be filtered out by the kidneys so they can deposit anywhere in the body and this is a potential health problem. For this reason, renal function is a concern for anyone receiving gadolinium injection. **Always follow your department's policy on administration of gadolinium!**

Why We Use Gad

TR, TE, and flip angle are methods to change tissue contrast on an image, but sometimes, no matter how hard we try, we just do not get the T1 contrast we want. GRE, T2, and STIR sequences are good but they may not be not good enough. When we look at images of various weightings, many questions are answered: Does it contain blood or blood products, is it fluid filled, is there more than one lesion? We know that there is some pathology there, but sometimes we just cannot make out the margins very well. Radiologists and, especially, surgeons want well defined margins whenever possible: Enter IV gadolinium. Administering IV contrast gives us another option for changing tissue contrast besides altering TRs, TEs, and flip angles.

We all knowingly say "Gadolinium shortens the T1 relaxation of a tissue," and we are correct. You may also know that it shortens the T2 relaxation as well but this chapter is not about that. We are just talking about the T1 relaxation that comes from gad.

How Does Gad Shorten the T1 of Tissues?

The body's reaction to an insult – trauma, infection, or tumor – is to force water (edema) to the area, and we know that edema has a long T1 relaxation time. On a T1 weighted image, the long T1 relaxing edema can be hard to see through to discern pathology. Contrast between tissues is low. Enter gadolinium. A gadolinium molecule has seven pairs of free electrons, and when gad is very close to water protons in a tissue there is an interaction. The reaction between the H_2O and gad electrons is termed a **proton–electron dipole interaction** or PEDI. A water proton interacts or binds to the gad molecule, gives off its energy, and releases from the gad. Another proton quickly takes its place, gives off its energy, then releases, and so on. A gad molecule can interact with multiple water protons at a time. This interaction facilitates an energy exchange between protons and electrons, allowing the energy received from the RF pulse to be released into the "lattice" at a **faster** than normal rate. Recall that T1 relaxation is sometimes called "spin-lattice relaxation." This interaction causes the tissues that soaked up the gad to be brighter than on the images taken prior to the administration of gad.

When different tissues T1 relax differently, they produce different amounts of signal at TE. When tissues have different signal intensity that is, and will always be, **image contrast**. This all sounds very impressive but what does it look like? The next few pages will show you.

Gad shortens the T1 of tissues and it will cross a non-intact blood–brain barrier (BBB). This happens all the time with tumors, infections, etc. Let's look at two sets of relaxation curves: Pre and post gad.

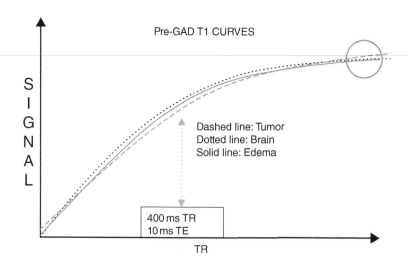

Figure 16.1 The "closeness" of the three curves tells us that all three tissues have very similar T1 relaxations and are difficult to distinguish from each other. You cannot tell them apart on a T1 weighted image.

Figure 16.1 shows the T1 relaxation curves of three different tissues. **The curves are very similar, meaning there is little T1 contrast between them.** The solid line is normal tissue, the dotted line is pathology, dashed line edema. The three tissues look very similar on a T1 weighted image. IV gad changes the T1 curve of the lesion (Figure 16.2).

Let's put this explanation together with pre and post gad images (Figures 16.3–16.5). Hopefully the previous explanation combined with these pictures will show how the theory translates into MR images.

Figure 16.5, bottom, clearly shows the mass (toxoplasmosis infection) vividly enhancing (T1 relaxation is markedly shortened) from the gad taken up out of the bloodstream due to breakdown of the BBB. Normal brain (with an intact BBB) does not enhance and the edema has no change in signal intensity as it has no blood supply. Edema is a reaction to the presence of the abnormal tissue, infection, or insult of some sort. The body's reaction to an "insult" is to force water to the area, hoping to dilute/wall off the insult.

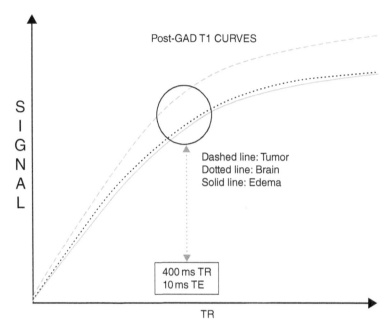

Post-GAD T1 CURVES

Dashed line: Tumor
Dotted line: Brain
Solid line: Edema

400 ms TR
10 ms TE

TR

Figure 16.2 T1 curves post gad. Tumor (dashed line) shows distinct shortening of T1 relaxation and will be brighter when compared to normal tissue (dotted line) and edema (solid line). The distance between tumor and brain curves has increased, indicating increased T1 contrast due to presence of gad (circled).

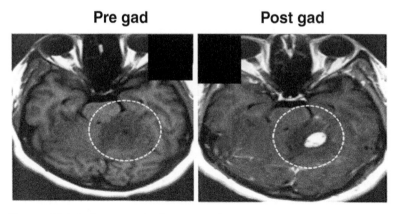

Pre gad   **Post gad**

Figure 16.3 Left, pre gad. There is pathology in the left cerebellum (known toxoplasmosis), but where is the mass in all that edema? Mass, edema, and brain all look very similar with no well-defined margins. Right, post gad.

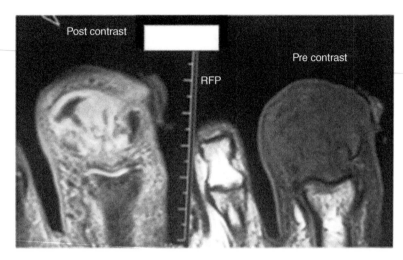

Figure 16.4 The first and second toes. Post gad image. The axial post gad image shows well-defined pathology.

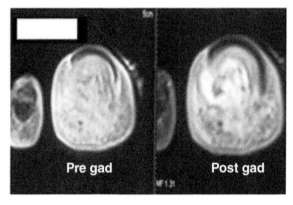

Figure 16.5 The first and second toes. Pre and post gad image. You know something is going on in the first toe (osteomyelitis) but not where. It is not well defined.

Gadolinium's Effect on T1 Relaxation

It is important to remember that when imaging post gad, you keep the TR short ($\approx$400–700 ms) to take full advantage of the T1 shortening effects of the gad. If you use too long a TR (circled on Figure 16.1) you will lose T1 contrast in general, but also diminish the effects of the gad.

As previously stated, gad, with its extra pairs of free electrons, accelerates T1 relaxation by helping the protons release their energy into the lattice. It is a quantum mechanics process where energy is exchanged.

All tissues have protons, but some have more than others. Pathologic tissue tends to have more protons per unit volume from rapid growth and angiogenesis (the rapid building of vasculature). The combination of a rich blood supply and rapid growth, when compared to normal tissue, pulls in more gad from the bloodstream. Consequently, abnormal tissue enhances more than normal tissue so will be brighter on post contrast sequences. Normal tissue picks up gad too (except in the brain), but not as much as abnormal tissue. This last statement repeats the vital concept of **image contrast. When there are signal intensity differences between tissues, for whatever reason, you have contrast.**

The Blood–Brain Barrier

The BBB is a semi-permeable border between the brain, circulating blood, and extracellular fluids. It is made up of densely packed endothelial cells and capillary walls. An intact BBB allows only certain molecules through by passive diffusion. Those select molecules are sugars, water, and amino acids to name a few. The BBB also acts to keep out pathogens and other large molecules from the CSF. The BBB keeps out 100% of large molecule drugs and about 97% of small molecule drugs. **This is why gad (a large molecule) does not cross an intact BBB.** There are several normal structures outside of the BBB that normally enhance: Optic nerves, choroid plexus, nasal mucosa, and pituitary and pineal glands.

The BBB becomes permeable (non-intact) in diseases like amyotrophic lateral sclerosis (AL, Lou Gehrig's disease), tumors, infection, trauma, or other causes of edema. Cancerous tissues excrete angiogenic proteins that increase vessel production,

affecting the permeability of vessels (BBB). In cases of inflam-
mation, the now permeable BBB allows phagocytes and anti-
biotics to pass, which is a good thing, but pathogens such as
toxoplasmosis, syphilis, and meningitis-causing streptococci can
also cross, and that is a bad thing. Liver failure can also affect
the function of the BBB.

There are times when the BBB is only slightly affected or
slightly permeable. High grade glioblastomas allow gad to pour
through the BBB and they enhance vividly, whereas low-grade
astrocytomas may not affect the BBB as much.

Your gadolinium brain protocol probably looks something
like this: DWI, T2 FLAIR, T2, GRE and T1 axials, inject,
and then post T1s. What follows is a slight alteration I have
seen in the past few years at multiple sites. Sequence order:
DWIs, pre T1s first, T2 FLAIR, **inject**, then do the T2 and
GREs, T2 Flair, followed by the post T1s. Gad does not affect
the tissue contrast of T2 FSE or GREs. It does a little bit on
the T2 FLAIR. More on this in a while. This "delay" I mentioned allows gad to get through a slightly permeable BBB
and into the lesion. The reason? With today's fast sequences
and scanners, your patient could, in theory, be walking out of
the department when the gad is just starting to cross into the
pathology. Multiple facilities have re-thought and re-ordered
their gad brain protocol.

A protocol change like this is something the radiologists need
to approve. It is just food for thought.

Post Contrast T2 FLAIR Imaging

"T2 FLAIR post gad?" "Aren't these sequences T2 weighted?"
"Isn't that why we call them T2 FLAIR?" Yes, yes, and yes.
On T2 FLAIR you will see some T1 weighting in the form of
the IV contrast. Remember I said early on in this book that all
images have some of all three weightings? It is just a matter
of which one dominates. **The twist is the TI.** Even though
we are suppressing the long T2 CSF with a long TI, it is that
fact itself that lets the gad be seen: The long TI lets short T1

tissue be seen. Pathology with enhancement on a T1 weighted sequence is also visible on a T2 FLAIR, not as vividly, but it is there. The T2 FLAIR sequence shows accumulated gad at low concentrations better than at higher concentrations. This means that if a lesion is only showing a little T1 enhancement you will probably see it better on the T2 FLAIR, partially because of the gad and also because the T2 FLAIR suppresses the surrounding edema. (Note on the word "concentrations". Here it means a lot of gad getting to the lesion, not a double or triple dose.) Vividly enhancing lesions do not show well on T2 FLAIR because of the T2 shortening effect of gad at high concentrations.

Post gad T2 FLAIRs can be used as "tie breaker" as it were. Is it enhancing or not?

Gad on T2 FLAIR is seen fairly well on structures outside of the BBB: Pituitary and pineal glands, choroid plexus, nasal mucosa, and turbinates (Figures 16.6–16.8).

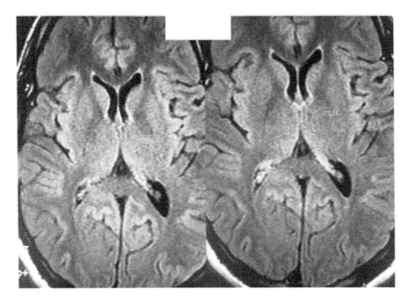

Figure 16.6 Same slice, same patient. T2 fat-sat FLAIRs pre and post gad at the level of the choroid plexus showing mild enhancement.

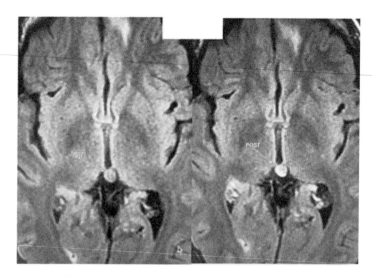

Figure 16.7 Same slice, same patient. At the level of the pineal gland, again showing enhancement from IV gad.

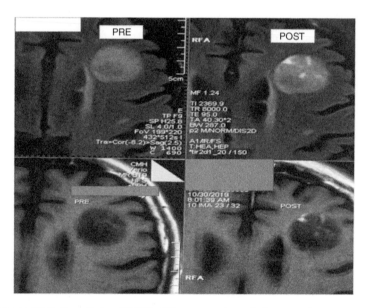

Figure 16.8 Top. Fat-sat T2 FLAIRs pre and post show gad enhancement inside a low-grade astrocytoma. Bottom. T1 FLAIR pre and post, again showing mild gadolinium enhancement. Both T2 FLAIR and T1s are same slice, same patient, with same window and level settings.

Blood vessels do not show any enhancement on the post gad T2 FLAIR images like they do on T1s because of high velocity signal loss (HVSL, flow void). This HVSL is due to the long TR/TEs on T2 FLAIR whereas T1s have shorter TR/TEs.

Imaging Gadolinium

Can you image gad? Nope. The gadolinium molecule is not imageable. It is a metal. Gad shortens the T1 of tissues so they get bright on a T1 image. It is the free electrons on the gad molecule interacting with hydrogen protons that makes some tissues bright.

Pure or straight gad out of the bottle is not imageable. You can try it if you like. Tape a bottle of gad to a phantom and try a T1. You'll get nothing (Figures 16.9 and 16.10).

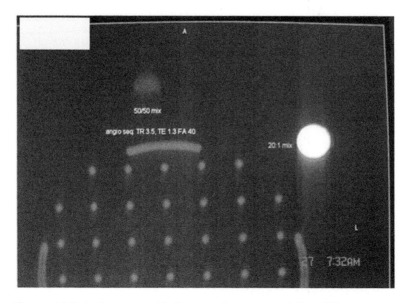

Figure 16.9 A phantom with three syringes containing different concentrations of gad and saline. On the left is pure gad in a syringe which you cannot even see, in the middle is a 50:50 mix, on the right is a 20:1. An MR angiogram sequence was run on this phantom for this demonstration.

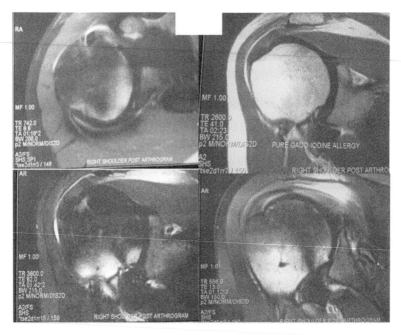

Figure 16.10 A set of images from a shoulder arthrogram in which pure gad was injected into the joint space. There was an iodine allergy. A T1 fat-sat, T2 fat-sat, and PD weighting are shown. Note that the intra-articular joint space is black because of pure gad. Fat-sat is incomplete/inhomogeneous on all views due to field inhomogeneity from the pure gad. Also note that the best image was the PD, again showing the joint space as black from lack of free water protons.

Gad is and can be seen on a CT scan. Gad, like iodine, is a heavy metal and both attenuate ionizing radiation. Due to its molecular structure, gad absorbs more radiation pound for pound compared to iodine. However, due to the usually low dose of gad given now for a typical MR exam when compared to the amount of iodine given for a typical CT scan, gad is only slightly seen on a CT scan. Visualization of gad is typically in the renal pelvis and urinary bladder. To see gad really well on a CT scan would require a dose of gad that would be toxic to the patient.

Years ago, back in the late 1990s and early 2000s, before NSF concerns, gad was administered in large doses to patients with

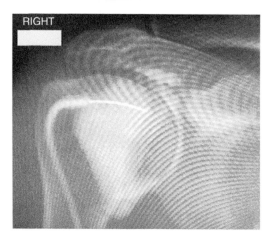

Figure 16.11 A shoulder radiograph/arthrogram using non-dilute gad. Gad is bright due to a high level of absorption of the x-ray beam. (Please excuse the zebra stripes, photo taken from a fluoroscopic monitor.)

severe allergies to iodine to take advantage of its radiopaque properties. This practice has now been abandoned due to NSF concerns. Some institutions have a 4-hour wait policy in between a gad MR and a CT scan. Figure 16.11 shows a radiograph of a shoulder arthrogram containing a combination of iodine and gadolinium.

Eovist®

Eovist or **gadoxetate disodium** (Bayer) is the only FDA-approved liver-specific **contrast** agent for MRI. It works like any other IV gadolinium-based contrast agent at first, meaning that it is seen and functions just like any other gadolinium-based contrast. The one major difference is that, unlike all other IV contrasts that are cleared from the body by glomerular filtration, Eovist is equally eliminated by both renal and hepatobiliary action. This means that the hepatocytes pick up the agent for elimination after a short delay of about 10–15 min. This lets the radiologist see what areas of the liver are filtering the agent,

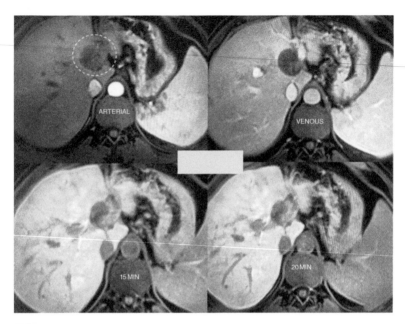

Figure 16.12 Top. Arterial and venous liver with Eovist. Bottom. 15- and 20-min delayed images. Pathology circled. Note that the liver is brighter than you would expect after such a long delay. Also note that the pathology is not enhancing, denoting that there are no working hepatocytes in the lesion. CT-guided biopsy found metastasis from colon cancer.

indicating that the hepatocytes are present and, more importantly, working. This is known as the hepatocyte phase and is where we do our typical 15- and 20-min delayed images. Being able to see where hepatocytes are working and where they are not can help determine/differentiate between focal nodular hyperplasia (FNH – a benign tumor of the liver) and hemangioma, or metastatic disease and hepatocellular carcinoma.

An Eovist liver study has the customary sequences to evaluate the liver – the routine arterial, venous, and delayed post contrast dynamic series – but because of the fact that the body clears Eovist through the liver (hepatobiliary excretion), there are typically 15- and 20-min delayed sequences to see the hepatocyte phases.

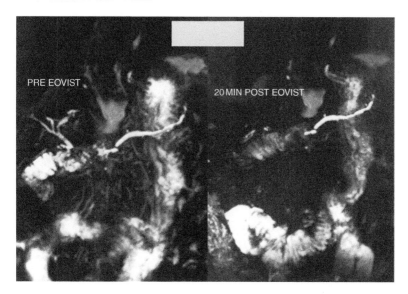

Figure 16.13 MRCP images taken pre and post injection of Eovist. As previously stated, Eovist is excreted mostly by the liver with a small percentage being excreted by the kidneys. Also remember that "straight" gad cannot be imaged. You cannot image metal. I had the opportunity to do an MRCP and Eovist liver combination. The Eovist is reconstituted by the liver and excreted in bile. Note the distinct loss of signal in the biliary tree on the post Eovist MRCP image, left. Also note that the pancreatic duct is maintained. While the pancreatic duct is part of the biliary tree, it does not receive bile output from the liver.

Your department will have a protocol for an Eovist liver scan. Be sure to follow your department's policy and protocol for administering Eovist.

Figures 16.12 and 16.13 show the different phases, together with some pre and post MRCP images showing the loss of signal in the biliary tree post injection.

Notes

Glossary

2D Sequence: When Fourier transform is applied in two directions – phase and frequency – for image production.

3D Sequence: Fourier transform is applied in three directions – slice, phase, and frequency. The third dimension in 3D comes from the slice select gradient, which is applied in a varying amplitude just like the PEG. This requires a third calculation for image processing, hence the name 3D.

Acceleration Factor: Relates to using a "parallel imaging" technique in order to scan faster. As the acceleration factor is made higher and higher, scan times are made shorter and shorter. Faster scan times come at the expense of signal to noise and resolution.

Acquisition/Nex/NSA: All three mean the same thing. They are vendor-specific terms for how many times the k-spaces are to be filled: 1, 2, or 3 times.

Active Shim: An electronic adjustment to the main magnetic field.

ADC Map: An extra set of images produced that shows an acute cerebrovascular accident (CVA) as dark. A corresponding area on the b-1000 should be bright.

Adiabatic: In thermodynamics, an adiabatic process is one in which no heat is lost or gained by a system. In MR, adiabatic RF pulses in an

MRI Physics: Tech to Tech Explanations, First Edition. Stephen J. Powers.
© 2021 John Wiley & Sons Ltd. Published 2021 by John Wiley & Sons Ltd.

Inversion Recovery sequence more precisely excite or invert (180°) tissues with less heating so SAR is less of a concern.

Aliasing (also known as Wrap or Fold-over): Happens when there is tissue outside of the field of view in the phase direction. Tissue outside the field of view is not sampled enough to satisfy the Nyquist Theorem and is mis-placed on the opposite side of the image.

Analog: In MRI, the echo that forms at TE is considered an "analog" signal. It is displayed or pictured as a continuously varying and physically decreasing sine wave. The array processor cannot work on a sine wave so the echo (a sine wave) is converted into numbers for conversion to the image.

Analog to Digital Converter (ADC): The signal received in the coil is analog. It is converted into numbers by the ADC.

Angiogenesis: A physiological process in which new blood vessels form/develop from pre-existing vessels, much like the root system of a plant that continues to develop. Angiogenesis is common in pathological tissues (tumors).

Anisotropic: When referring to a pixel, if the pixel is not square (e.g.1 mm × 1 mm), then the pixel is anisotropic.

Annifact Artifact: Artifact caused by signal from outside of the field of view due to having too many coils turned on.

Arterial Spin Labeling (ASL): A proton density weighted sequence that can give perfusion-like information without an injection of IV gadolinium-based contrast. It gives the relative cerebral blood flow (rCBV) for an area of interest.

Artifact: An area or point in the image(s) that contains false information or data. There are many causes of image artifacts, as outlined in Chapter 12. FYI: All images have artifact(s) of some sort from some cause or reason. Artifacts cannot be eliminated; they can only be minimized/lessened.

Axial Plane (also known as the "Z" plane): Assuming the patient is head first and supine, axial slices transect the patient from head to toe.

b-Value or b-Factor: In diffusion weighted imaging, the "b" value is relative to the **strength and/or duration** of the diffusion gradients being applied for the sequence. The higher or greater the b-value, the more sensitive the sequence is to decrease cellular diffusion. For example, a 500 b-value is less sensitive to a stroke in the brain than is a 1000 b-value.

B_0: The main magnetic field. it is also known as the longitudinal field, and sometimes termed "B-naught" (naught = zero). It is also called the Z axis.

B_0 **(image):** In DWI, image acquired without DW gradients applied. Basically, low-resolution T2 weighted images.

B_1: The RF field applied for slice selection and refocusing. The RF flips the protons into the transverse plane.

Bandwidth (B/W): In MRI, bandwidth is a range of frequencies. There are two different bandwidths: Receiver B/W, which is taken while sampling the echo; and Transmitter B/W, which is a range of frequencies that excites a slice.

Big Three (The): Local and main magnetic field inhomogeneities, and magnetic susceptibility.

Bird Cage Coil: A coil type similar to a saddle coil where the anatomy is placed inside of the coil for imaging. It may slide over the anatomy or close over the top.

Black Blood: An SE sequence with an RF pulse specifically used to make blood appear black on the images. A similar effect is often seen on CSE sequences where the blood has moved out of the slice and been replaced by "unexcited" blood. Unexcited tissue cannot give signal. This effect is often referred to as a "flow void."

Blood Brain Barrier (BBB): A semi-permeable matrix of tissues and fibers that only lets certain molecules and drugs into the brain. Gadolinium is one such molecule that **will not cross** an intact BBB. Pathology such as tumors and infection will make the BBB a less effective barrier and will allow gadolinium to cross and be taken up by the abnormality.

Body Coil: Typically refers to the large "inherent" or internal transmit/receive RF transmitting coil located inside the bore of the scanner.

Bound Protons: A group or pool of protons that are tightly bound/attached to another molecule and are not able to be "flipped" by an RF pulse. They will not give any signal at TE. Hydrogen protons in cortical bone, tendons, or ligaments are bound.

Brownian Movement or Motion: An erratic/random movement of microscopic particles that results in collisions with other molecules in a surrounding medium. In other words, water and other intracellular chemicals are moving within, into, and out of the cell. Equate this to "bumper cars" at an amusement park. If the cells are perfused, there is energy to move around; if they are not perfused, the energy is shut off and the bumper cars stop moving.

Cartesian Coordinates: The X, Y, Z coordinate system of localization. It is used to locate a point relative to a fixed reference. In MR, that fixed reference is isocenter, whose coordinates are 0, 0, and 0. The coordinates specify each point along a plane as set by numerical coordinates, which are assigned distances along the three fixed perpendicular planes.

Cellular Respiration: A process in which cells combine oxygen and nutrient molecules and use the chemical energy from these substances to perform activities such as discarding waste products, carbon dioxide, and water.

Center Frequency (CF): The precessional frequency of the center slice of a stack or slab.

Center Lines (of k-space): Those lines in the middle or center portion of k-space. The center 25% of lines in k-space contribute close to 90% of an image's contrast.

Centric k-Space Filling: A filling scheme that fills the center lines first for maximum image contrast. The outer lines are filled last. This scheme is often used in contrast MRA or dynamic imaging studies.

Cerebral Spinal fluid (CSF): Fluid surrounding the brain and spinal cord. It has the highest PD of all human tissue as it is mostly water. Urine is a close second.

Chemical Saturation or "Chem Sat": When a specific chemical (tissue) like fat or water is targeted with RF pulses to not give signal at TE. A fancy name for fat-sat.

Chemical Shift: The frequency difference between fat and water.

Chemical Shift Artifact: An artifact seen in the frequency direction. A black border is seen on one side of a structure, a white border on the other. It is caused by narrow receiver B/Ws. There are really two kinds of chemical shift artifact. The first is chemical shift as described above. The second kind is also known as the OOP echo, where there is a black line around all tissues in both the phase and frequency directions.

Cine Loop: A series of MR images acquired rapidly and repeatedly like an MR movie. Also known as "real-time."

Circle of Willis (COW): The major "cross roads" of connections for all the major arteries supplying blood to the brain. It is comprised of the anterior, middle, and posterior cerebral arteries.

Coil(s): A generic term in MR for a loop or loops of wires that collect the signal produced at the TE. Some coils are designed for very specific purposes or more general imaging.

Collapsed Images: All scanners produce these. When an MRA sequence has finished running, a set of images, usually an anterior/posterior (A/P), superior/inferior (S/I), and right/left (R/L), are processed by the scanner. Collapsed means that all the slices or locations are projected as one image. You might say that they are stacked up onto one another as if you were looking at all the data at once. It is a quick way to check image quality in the form motion and coverage. These images are truly the "MIPs" (MIP" stands for maximum intensity projection). Basically, it is showing you all the bright pixels (maximum intensity) in one projection. See "Maximum Intensity Projection" for more information.

Concatenations (Acquisitions): A number that is input to allow you to use a lower TR to maintain image contrast. It can let you halve the TR. It can also be used to shorten a breath-hold in chest/abdomen/pelvis studies. Example: 30 slices needs 1000 ms to acquire at 1 concat, but 2 concats lets you use a 500 TR. Fifteen slices are acquired in 500 TR, the other 15 slices in another 500 TR. In another example, a 42 s breath-hold at 1 acquisition becomes two 21 s breath-holds with 2 acquisitions.

Conjugate Symmetry of k-Space: There is symmetry or redundancy in k-space which is a fundamental property for Fourier transformation. Basically, one only needs half the data to characterize any place in k-space. This means that if there is a +2X3Y data point, then because of the symmetry in k-space there will be a -2X3Y data point. This symmetry can be taken advantage of to fill lines of k-space without actually scanning them.

Contrast: A difference in signal intensities between tissues.

Contrast Enhanced MRA (CE-MRA): IV contrast is injected, and data acquisition is timed to contrast reaching the target vessel(s).

Contrast to Noise Ratio (CNR): Amount of contrast over the level of noise.

Contrast Triangle: A visual depiction of the three different topics or concerns to that contribute to image quality: Contrast, signal to noise, and resolution.

Conventional Spin Echo (CSE): 90°, 180°, followed by an echo.

Corduroy Artifact: Artifact resulting from a single or multiple "spike" (abnormally high signal amplitudes) in the data causing the classic "corduroy" look to the image. There are several causes of these "spikes."

Coronal Plane: Assuming the patient is head first and supine, the coronal plane transects the patient A/P. The "Y" direction.

Cross-Excitation: Often used synonymously with cross-talk. Cross-excitation happens when two or more slices cross each other. The common tissue of the slices is seen as dark as the common tissue has not had time to T1 relax and is actually saturated to a point. This artifact is commonly seen posterior to the cord in lumbar spine images.

Cross-Talk: This artifact was more common many years ago. Basically, the RF profile of one slice had some RF in common with the slice next to it. Slice A would excite a little bit of slice B, signal in slice B was a little bit less. Slice B excited a little bit of slice C and so on. Putting a gap between slices is the most common way to eliminate this artifact.

Cryogen: A substance capable of producing very low temperature(s).

dB/dT: Rate of change (d) of a magnetic field (B) over change (d) in time (t). This indicates how fast the gradient field changes over time.

Decay Curve: A T2 curve. A graph depicting a number or volume of protons that have left (de-phased) the X/Y plane over a given time. Typically, two curves are shown in order to compare a fast-decaying tissue against a lower decaying tissue. Protons will stay together (be in phase) in the X/Y for only

a short period of time. Signal quickly begins to decay. See also "Relaxation Curve."

De-phasing: The act of protons getting out of sync with each other. The direction of de-phasing is a function of the main magnetic field. De-phasing can be recovered by two methods: A 180° refocusing RF pulse or a magnetic gradient application.

Diamagnetic: A substance with no permanent magnetic dipole such as water, nickel, or bismuth, that, in the presence of an external magnetic field, sets up an opposite magnetic field to that of the external field. This means it is mildly repulsed by a magnetic field. Diamagnetic substances have unpaired electrons, which is the opposite of "paramagnetic" substances that have unpaired electrons. Gadolinium is a paramagnetic material.

Dielectric Effect or Standing Wave Artifact: This is often seen at 3 T but it can happen at any field strength. It is related to the wavelength of the RF at 3 T having a propensity to "bounce back" or echo out. One RF is bouncing back out while a second is coming into the anatomy. They cancel each other out, causing the classic area of signal loss. Two waves are existing at the same time, hence the name "standing wave."

Diethylenetriamine pentaacetate (DTPA): A chelating agent with multiple uses in metal-containing diagnostic agents such as MRI contrast agents, and nuclear medicine scanning. It is a synthetic compound that can sequester (bind to) metal ions and form highly stable DTPA–metal ion complexes. Bonding to the gadolinium molecule makes it too large to get through an intact BBB, but big enough to be taken out of the blood stream by glomerular filtration.

Diffusion: At the cellular level, the act of a cell moving nutrients, waste, and water in and/or out through its membrane. Diffusion requires energy in the form of a blood supply to the tissue.

Diffusion Weighted Imaging (DWI): An echo planar type of sequence where the image contrast comes from differences in tissue diffu-

sion. DW imaging is a staple sequence in brain imaging for stroke.

Digital to Analog Converter (DAC): The RF pulse instruction from the computer to the Radio Frequency Power Amplifier (RFPA) is numeric. The DAC converts numbers to analog so the RFPA can transmit the RF. This works opposite to the way the ADC works. They do not oppose each other; they just have two separate and different jobs.

Dixon Method or Technique: A method of producing fat-sat images at low field strengths. It has recently become popular at high fields. An IP and OOP echo are acquired and mathematically manipulated to produce four different contrasts: IP, OOP, fat, and water images.

Driven Equilibrium (DE, also known as DRIVE): This uses an extra $+180°$ then a $-90°$ set of RF pulses at the end of the echo train to force, drive, or accelerate T1 relaxation.

Duty Cycle: A statement on gradient performance that is sequence dependent. It is a percentage of time that the gradients are able to work at their maximum strength. A 95–100% duty cycle is to be expected in most of the modern high field scanners.

Dynamic Susceptibility of Contrast (DSC, also known as Perfusion): DSC is often performed in the brain to aid in the planning of treatment for a stroke or CVA. It requires a rapid injection of IV contrast with repeated rapid sets of images of the brain. That is the **"dynamic"** part. The **susceptibility** part is taking advantage of the "metallic" properties of the contrast as it reaches the brain. As the gadolinium reaches and "perfuses" the brain, signal in the brain will decrease. Portions that are not perfused will not decrease in signal. Tissues that are not being perfused very well will take longer to decrease in signal. DCS studies show which tissues are either perfused, not perfused, or poorly perfused. See also "Perfusion Weighted Imaging." **Terms associated with DSC or perfusion studies include:**

- **Mean Transit Time (MTT):** The **average** (mean) time it takes for the contrast to reach (wash in) and exit (wash out) the region of interest (ROI). Basically: How long does the gadolinium hang around in the tissue?

- **Time to Peak (TTP):** The time it takes for the gadolinium bolus to reach its highest concentration, causing maximum signal loss in the ROI.

- **Relative Cerebral Blood Flow (rCBF):** A red, yellow, and blue colored map showing red as high flow, yellow less, and blue even less flow. Important in stroke evaluation, it is a qualitative representation of the amount of blood flow in the tissue.

- **Relative Cerebral Blood Volume (rCBV):** A similar color map as in rCBF and used most often in tumor evaluation/characterization. It is a qualitative representation of the amount of blood in the tissue.

Echo (also known as the TE): Where a signal is induced

in the coil by the effects of a refocusing mechanism.

Echo Planar Imaging: An imaging technique where a complete "planar" image (slice) is obtained with one selective excitation pulse.

Echo Spacing (ES): The time in ms (milliseconds) in between echo formation. Typically, the first TE (the minimum TE) is also the echo spacing. Echo spacing in spin echo sequences is about 10 ms or lower. A low ES is desirable to decrease blurring. Factors affecting ES are: FOV, receiver B/W, and frequency matrix.

Echo Train Balancing: The ideal of "echo train balancing" is to have the effective TE be the center or middle echo of the echo train. This will place the effective TEs in the center of k-space for the best image contrast.

Echo Train Length (ETL): In turbo or fast spin echo imaging, multiple echoes are produced during the sequence. The number of echoes can vary from as low as two to 24 or even more. The number of echoes produced is called the ETL. The ETL has an effect on image contrast. Short ETLs are used for T1 weighted imaging with an ETL of 2–4, while T2 weighted contrast images often have an ETL of 18–24 or more. The more echoes, the more T2 contrast is placed into the k-space. RF exposure (SAR) increases with longer ETLs.

Effective TE (ETE): In fast or turbo spin echo sequences multiple echoes are produced per TR. The echo chosen for the image contrast is said to be the "effective TE". The effective TEs will be placed in the center lines of k-space during the run of the sequence.

Elliptical Centric k-Space Filling: In MRA sequences, the center lines are filled in an outwardly spiraling direction starting from the center and moving outward.

Equilibrium: A state or condition of a "system" in which all parts have the same temperature. Equilibrium occurs in MR, when, over a sufficient amount of time (ms), the tissues have released all of their RF energy into the lattice.

Ernst Angle: A flip angle that produces the maximum

signal in a tissue for a particular TR. At a constant TR (e.g. 500 ms), SNR increases with higher and higher flip angles, but only to a point. At a certain flip angle, the Ernst Angle, tissue starts to saturate (not enough time to T1 relax) and signal begins to decrease. Ernst Angle sequences are more often used at 3 T than at 1.5 T. This is because SAR is a concern at 3 T and getting good T1 contrast can also be a challenge at 3 T. Ernst Angle sequences can give better T1 contrast than conventional SE sequences.

Estimated Glomerular Filtration Rate (eGFR): See "Glomerular Filtration Rate" for additional information

Excitation Pulse: The initial application of RF to push the longitudinal NMV to a certain angle into the transverse, e.g. 90° for a SE, or 20° for a GRE. **Note:** The RF pulse does not have a "flip angle" in it; the amount of "flip" or "tip" is a function of the amount of time the RF is applied. **A 180° pulse means the RF is applied for twice as long as it was for a 90°.** Excitation is sometimes symbolized as: α.

Exponential ADC Map (eADC Map): In DWI imaging, a calculated image set used to further exclude T2 shine through. The calculation is the B_0 divided by (÷) the DWI image.

Faraday Cage: Copper lining in the ceiling, walls, and floor of the scan room to keep external RF out and the RF transmitted during a sequence in the scan room.

Faraday's Law of Induction: A law of physics where a magnetic field moving through or past a conductor will induce current in that conductor.

Fast Fourier Transform (FFT): A numerical algorithm to compute a discrete Fourier transform for a sequence. Fourier transform converts signals from their original form into a representation in the frequency domain. It breaks down a group of frequencies into the individual frequencies.

Fast Spin Echo (FSE) or Turbo Spin Echo (TSE): A variation on the spin echo pulse sequence where multiple echoes (more than one), called an echo train, are produced per TR in order to decrease scan time. Scan time decreases as a function of the ELT.

Fast Spoiled Gradient Recalled (FSPGR): The FSPGR sequence uses an RF pulse to "spoil" residual transverse net magnetization vectors. Hear SPGR, think T1 weighted GRE.

Fast Recovery, Drive, or Driven Equilibrium: In spin echo and FSE imaging, there will be some residual transverse net magnetization (long T2 tissue vectors). Given enough time, these vectors will relax equilibrium on their own. This, though, takes time. Fast recovery or DRIVE uses negative polarity RF pulses to force or drive the vectors back to longitudinal.

Fat Saturation (fat-sat, F/S): There are several methods to decrease signal from fat-containing tissue. Fat-sat uses RF pulses **specifically tuned to the precessional frequency of fat** which are applied at the beginning of the pulse sequence. Consequently, fat has received multiple RF pulses and is rendered unable to give much signal at TE. Often abbreviated as F/S or FS.

Fat Suppression: As in a STIR sequence, signal from fat is suppressed by the application of an inversion pulse, waiting an appropriate amount of time in ms (the TI) before beginning the pulse sequence. The affect is that fat (and other short T1 relaxing tissues) is able to give very little signal at TE.

Ferrous: Containing a percentage of iron and so forcibly attracted to a magnet (**non-ferrous** means having little to no iron content and not attracted by a magnet). Common ferrous materials are hair pins (bobby pins and paper clips). These common objects can and will be pulled into the scanner. MR-safe wheelchairs are made of "non-ferrous" material such as aluminum which is not attracted to a magnet.

Field of View (FOV): Analogous to the film size in x-ray, this is the area to be scanned in the slice select direction. It is assumed to be square (200 mm × 200 mm or 20 cm × 20 cm) unless otherwise stated as in a rectangular FOV. The FOV is a function of or comes from the FEG. A smaller FOV can cause the minimum TE to increase slightly. A small FOV needs a strong application of the FEG.

Flip Angle (F/A): The angle or degrees away from longitudinal the NMV achieves from an RF pulse. This is a function of time that the RF is turned on. See "Excitation Pulse." F/A can also be a function of the strength or amplitude of the RF application. A stronger pulse flips the protons over faster, which may allow a shortening of the TR and or the TE.

Flow Compensation (Flow Comp, also known as Gradient Motion Refocusing (GMR) or Gradient Motion Nulling (GMN): A series of gradient applications applied before TE to compensate for loss of signal from flow, or to reduce pulsatile artifacts.

Flow Related Enhancement: A newer term used interchangeably with TOF MRA. Think of it this way: The vessel's **enhancement** is **related** to its **flow**.

Flow Types: Flowing blood can be categorized or described by four basic types:

laminar = normal; vortex = jet like; turbulent = tumbling; and finally, stagnant = very slow to not flowing at all.

Flow Void: A very commonly used description of a lack of signal in a blood vessel(s). This is meant to state/indicate that the lack of signal in a vessel is due to flowing blood. This is synonymous with high velocity signal loss (HVSL). Both of these terms indicate that excited blood has moved out of the slice before the TE.

For example: On CSE and FSE sequences where blood has moved out of the slice it is replaced by "unexcited "blood at the TE. Unexcited tissue cannot give signal. This effect is often referred to as a "flow void."

Fluid Attention Inversion Recovery (FLAIR): A variation on a spin echo sequence used in the brain and spine to suppress signal from CSF.

Fold-over: Another name or term for the artifact wrap.

Fourier Transform: An algorithm used to divide or separate the frequency components of an echo from its various amplitudes as a function over time. Fourier transform is vital to all modalities, and especially in MRI. Signals received by coils in MRI are a complex of periodic signals made up of a large number of different frequencies (the bandwidth). Fourier transform represents/breaks down data over its frequency axis. An MR spectroscopy image is a simple example in which different molecules are at different frequencies along an axis.

Fractional Echo or Partial Echo: When only part of or a fraction of the echo is sampled at TE. Most often this is done when acquiring a CE-MRA sequence in order to save time (shorten the TR).

Free Induction Decay (FID): A signal generated by the excitation RF pulse.

Free Protons: Protons that are not tightly affixed to another structure or molecule. They are "free" to be flipped by an excitation pulse and can therefore contribute to the signal at TE. Almost all protons in the body are "free," examples are those in muscle, liver, brain, and bone marrow. See also "Bound Protons."

Frequency: This has more than one meaning in MRI. Frequency as related to RF is the number of times something repeats or occurs in a given period of time.

It can also be referred to as "temporal frequency." Temporal is an adjective relating to "time". Radiofrequency (RF) is measured by units of Hertz (Hz). This is equal to one occurrence, oscillation, or repetition per second. Megahertz (MHz), means Million Hertz or million repeats. 63 MHz is 63 million oscillations per second.

Frequency Direction: One of the three cardinal directions in MRI. The other two are phase and slice.

Frequency Encoding: This happens after the refocusing event. As the protons rephase, the FEG is applied while the echo is sampled.

Frequency Encoding Gradient (FEG): Gradient applied during the TE. Sometimes symbolized by ν (nu).

Frequency Matrix: The number of pixels in the scan matrix in the frequency direction. This is also the number of times the echo is sampled. A higher frequency matrix may cause the TE to lengthen. Remember that the more work is asked of the scanner (more frequency encodes), the more time it will take. In this case, asking for more samples of the echo, the FEG has to be left on for a longer period of time.

Fringe Field: In MR, a weaker surrounding magnetic field that gets stronger as one gets closer to the scanner/bore. The equivalent to "scatter radiation" in x-ray.

Gadolinium: A rare earth metal with seven unpaired electrons that help protons lose energy (T1 relax) that was acquired from the RF pulses. Gadolinium is considered "paramagnetic" because of the unpaired electrons.

Gamma: Term for the gyromagnetic ratio of hydrogen. Symbol: γ.

Gauss: A unit of magnetic strength where 10,000 G = 1 Tesla (T).

Generalized Auto Calibrating Partially Parallel Acquisition (GRAPPA): A parallel imaging method in which the center lines of k-space are fully sampled while the outer lines are "under-sampled," thus saving time. There is a slight loss in resolution with this method.

Ghosting Artifact: A vague repeated duplication of a structure in the phase direction. It is caused by repetitive motion from the heart, or respirations. It is a motion artifact but should not be confused with gross patient motion.

Gibbs Artifact: Commonly substituted with truncation, Gibbs artifact commonly comes from extremely aniso-tropic pixels. If the phase matrix is less than half the frequency matrix, Gibbs arti-fact will occur. See also "Ringing Artifact."

Glomerular Filtration Rate (GFR): A number that indi-cates how well a patient's kidneys are working (or if they are failing). The esti-mated (eGFR) calculation that is performed uses the factors of age, gender, race, and a current serum creati-nine. The "e" means it is an estimate, which also means there can be a significant margin for error.

Glutamate/Glutamine (Peaks): Glutamate and

glutamine are two brain metabolites and indicate neuronal transmitters.

Gradient: A gradient is a hill. In MRI it indicates an "magnetic hill" that is high (strong) on one side, and weak on the other.

Gradient Echo or Gradient Recalled Echo (GRE): One of the two pulse sequences in MRI. It is characterized by an excitation pulse without a refocusing pulse. It uses a gradient pulse to refocus the protons.

Gradient Magnetic Fields: These are time varying magnetic fields applied to the static magnetic field. They temporarily and selectively change the strength of the main magnetic field.

Gradient Warp: When imaging at the edge of a gradient uniformity, the image is seen as warping or bending. Gradients need to be linear, constant, and reproducible. Imaging out near the end of a gradients limit for linearity is where the IQ starts to suffer.

Grey Matter (GM): The more superficial layer of brain tissue that contains mostly nerve cell bodies and few myelinated fibers and therefore appears grey on dissection. Compare with "White Matter."

Gyromagnetic ratio (GMR): A mathematical constant in the Larmor Equation. Its value is 42.57 MHz for hydrogen at 1 T. See "Larmor Equation."

Half Fourier: Uses k-space symmetry to interpolate data points and fill k-space faster. Is also called complex conjugate symmetry.

Half Fourier Acquired Single Shot Turbo Spin Echo (HASTE): Half of the data is acquired with one excitation pulse, the other half with a second RF excitation pulse. Basically, the two single shots are then interleaved or combined.

Hard Shim: Shimming is used to make something level. In MRI to shim is make the magnetic field uniform. A hard shim is a permanent adjustment to the field via small pieces of aluminum attached inside the bore.

Helium (He: An inert (not flammable) naturally occurring gaseous element.

Helmholtz Coil: A pair of coils designed to generate a

uniform signal from the tissue in between them.

High Velocity Signal Loss (HVSL): Lack of signal in a vessel due to moving (flowing) blood. Excited blood has moved out of the slice before the 180° and gives no signal at TE. Synonymous with, or used instead of, "Flow Void."

Hunter's Angle: A term used when speaking about spectroscopy. Dr Hunter, a neurologist, would look at a spectroscopy, and if a line drawn from the N-acetyl aspartate (NAA) peak to the creatine-choline peaks was about 45°, that spectroscopy was likely normal.

Image Quality (IQ): An image with good tissue contrast, SNR, and resolution is said to have good "image quality or IQ." Other aspects of good image quality can include being free of artifacts and well positioned to demonstrate the desired anatomy.

In Phase (IP): There are two definitions: **1:** In a GRE sequence when the **TE** is at a time in ms when the fat and water vectors point in the same direction, thus adding up to make the overall SNR higher. This is opposed by the out of phase (OOP) TE when vectors point in opposite directions. Signal will drop. **2:** When protons of all tissues are all pointing in the same direction they are said to be "in phase."

In-Phase Echo: An "in-phase" echo is when both fat and water vectors are pointing in the same direction within a pixel. They combine their signal and the pixel(s) becomes brighter.

In-Plane Saturation: In an MRA sequence, this refers to the loss of signal from blood due to the blood flowing in the slice or slab (the plane) for too long. That blood has received many RF pulses and begins to "saturate" just like the background tissue. Contrast between the vessel and the background is lost.

Internal Auditory Canal/ Internal Auditory Meatus (IACs/IAMs): The foramen in the petrous portion of the sphenoid bone from which the seventh and eighth cranial nerves exit.

Inversion: When a set of vectors is flipped or inverted from its original position (e.g. 0° flipped to 180°) by an RF pulse.

Inversion Pulse: Usually a 180° RF pulse that flips the NMV halfway around. Vector ↑ gets hit with a 180° and becomes vector ↓ as a STIR or FLAIR sequence.

Inversion Recovery (IR): A pulse sequence that allows suppression of tissues by varying the TI in the sequence. See "Inversion Time." An inversion recovery sequence contains three RF pulses: 180°, 90°, and 180°. TIs or inversion times, measured in milliseconds (ms), can be changed from short to long depending on which tissue is to be suppressed.

IR Prep: An 180° (inversion) RF pulse (or pulses) is applied in order to "prep" tissue(s) to either enhance or suppress signals from certain tissues by varied TIs. If you think about it, STIR and FLAIR can be considered IR prepped sequences. If the base sequence is a 3D Spoiled Gradient Echo (SPGR), the TI can be varied to enhance Grey/White Matter (GM/WM) differentiation or actually suppress WM to increase tissue conspicuity between WM and multiple sclerosis (MS) plaques.

Isotropic: When referring to a pixel, if the pixel or voxel is square (e.g. $1 \times 1 \times 1$ mm), then the pixel/voxel is isotropic.

J-Coupling: A quantum mechanics interaction between nuclear spins within the same molecule. A full explanation is beyond the scope of this book. In short, J coupling is responsible for the modulation (multiplication) of the signal of fat during a fast spin echo sequence.

k-Space: A temporary storage area for image data (raw data) prior to image processing. k Is an arithmetic symbol that denotes frequency. A k-space is an imaginary entity that you cannot touch or see. It is a space to store "ks" or "frequencies. There is one k-space per slice for that slice's raw data. There are multiple ways or methods to fill k-space.

Lactate: A metabolite found in the brain. It is displayed on a spectroscopy image and is a marker of cellular death.

Laminar Flow: In a blood vessel, normal undisturbed or unobstructed flow of blood.

Larmor Equation: The equation used to find the precessional frequency of hydrogen at any field strength: Wo $= \gamma B_0$ where Wobble (Wo) or frequency, γ is the gyromagnetic ratio of hydrogen at 1 T. This number is a constant. B_0 is the field strength of the magnet for which you are trying to find the precessional frequency. Example: Wo $= 42.57 \times B_0$; Wo $= 42.57 \times 0.75$ T; Wo $= 31.91$ MHz.

Larmor Frequency: The precessional frequency (PF) of hydrogen at 1 T $= 42.57$ MHz.

Lattice: The local environment to which protons give off or exchange energy in longitudinal relaxation. See "T1" relaxation.

Linear Filling of k-Space: A k-space filling method that fills one line at a time. It is less efficient time-wise than the method used in fast/turbo spin echo.

Logical Gradients: The X, Y, and Z gradients do the three jobs of spatial encoding. Each one can do any job, but which one will do which job? This is the thinking or logical portion.

Longitudinal Magnetization: The net magnetization vector (NMV) that runs along the static magnetic field or Z direction. Its counterpart is the transverse NMV.

Longitudinal Plane: The north/south direction of the magnet. The B_0 or Z plane.

Magic Angle Artifact: An artifact sometimes seen on T1 and PD weighted images. If a tendon is positioned at approximately 55° to B_0 and with a short TE, then high signal can be seen on the tendon mimicking pathology.

Magnetic Resonance Spectroscopy (MRS): A sequence that allows a determination of the concentration of different metabolites in a specific region of interest. Different disease processes have different concentrations of metabolites.

Magnetic Susceptibility: A measure of a tissue' or substance's ability to be magnetized. Air cannot be magnetized whereas soft tissues can be magnetized.

Magnetization Prepared (MP, or Mag Prepped): The use of an RF pulse before the start of a sequence in order to either null signal from a tissue or to enhance a tissue's contrast.

Magnetization Transfer (MT): A technique with an off-center RF pulse used to decrease the signal from a tissue, thus increasing conspicuity of another. Very commonly used in brain MRAs to decrease signal from the background white matter, thus brightening blood vessels.

Main Magnetic Field (MMF): Also known as B_0.

Matrix: A term to describe the resolution of an image. The matrix is an array of rows and columns, each having a direction: Phase and frequency. A scan matrix of 256×256 (256^2) means that there are 256 pixels in both the phase and frequency directions. Pixel size is determined by the FOV and the scan matrix.

Maximum Intensity Projection (MIP, also known as Collapsed Images): We all call the "cut-outs" we do of the vessels from an MRA data set an "MIP". They are not. That is a misnomer. "Cut-outs" is a bit more accurate, but "MIPs" is and what has been used for a long time so that is what we call them. Scanners have post-processing programs that allow us to "cut out" or remove background/low-signal intensity structures from MRA data sets to better see blood vessels. You want to see just the "maximum intensity" (bright pixels) structures (i.e. the blood vessels. See "Collapsed Images" for more information.

Metabolites: Chemicals that are produced in the brain as a result of cellular activity. Normal brain tissue has a certain amount/level of the various metabolites. Metabolite levels will change (raise/lower) in the presence of different disease processes or conditions.

Metal Artifact: Metal inside the FOV causes the precessional frequencies to drift off the center frequency determined by the scanner during pre-scan. This, in turn, causes an area to be unable to be imaged.

Metal Artifact Reduction Series or Sequence (MARS): A generic non-vendor-specific term for adjusting a sequence's scan parameters to lessen the metal artifact in the images. Any scanner can be adjusted to scan with this series of parameter adjustments. Factors adjusted are: Echo train length, receiver B/W, and TE.

Minimum Intensity Projection (Min. IP): A post processing program used to display or project pixels with the **least** or **minimum signal intensity**, usually blood vessels. It is used in reformatting 3D susceptibility weighted images or sequences. These sequences are specifically done looking for presence of blood or petechial hemorrhage post trauma or post operatively.

Minimum TE (Min. TE): The shortest possible TE obtainable after excitation and refocusing. There are several scan factors that can affect the Min. TE such as the FOV, frequency matrix, slice thickness, and receiver B/W.

Moiré Fringe Artifact: Artifact caused by several things on a steady state GRE sequence, usually from wrap combining with magnetic field inhomogeneities, especially at the edge of the FOV.

Motion Artifact: Artifact always seen in the phase direction because the phase direction is encoded many times during the course of the sequence, causing the associated "smearing" in the phase direction.

Multiple Overlapping Thin Section Angiography (MOTSA): In MRAs, having blood in the slice or slab for as short a time as possible in order to minimize in-plane saturation. To lessen the effects of in-plane saturation, several thin slabs or sections are positioned so that they overlap. Overlap is vital. You do not want to miss any of the vessel.

Multi-shot: When multiple TRs are required to fill a *k*-space for a slice. This is what is being done for the vast majority of imaging in MR. See also "Single Shot."

Nephrogenic Systemic Fibrosis (NSF): A possible consequence of the breakdown of the bonds between the gadolinium molecule and its chelating agent, leading to free gadolinium radicals being released into the body. Fibrous tissue can form in multiple locations in the body related to the reaction to the presence of gadolinium.

Net Magnetization Vector (NMV): The sum of many small vectors adding up into a larger vector.

Nex/NSA/Acq: Vendor-specific terms or acronyms stating the number of times each *k*-space will be filled (e.g. 2 "nex" means that each line is filled twice before filling the next line, example: Line 1 is filled twice, then line 2 gets filled twice, followed by line 3 being filled twice).

Noise: Something that is present in all electronic equipment. It is low-level meaningless random signal that detracts from image quality. It is the second factor in the signal to noise ratio equation. Ideally there is more signal received by the coils than there is noise.

Non-Cartesian: Describes *k*-space filling. Cartesian filling is "line by line" and has been the most common method for filling *k*-space since MRI began 30 or more years ago. In the last 10–15 years, other methods of filling *k*-space have evolved and are in wide use. Some of these other non-cartesian methods include elliptical centric (spiral), radial (blade like), and rectilinear, common in EPI sequences.

Non-Ferrous: A quality of a metal meaning that it contains little to no iron and thus is not attracted towards a magnetic field.

No Phase Wrap (GE), Phase Oversampling (Siemens), Fold-over suppression (Philips): Sequence options to eliminate or minimize the artifact called wrap, aliasing, or fold-over.

Null Point: A term referenced when describing IR sequences. The null point is determined by multiplying a tissue's T1 relaxation time by 0.69. This math determines what TI to use to suppress signal from a tissue. For example, the T1 relaxation of fat is approximately 230 ms at 1.5 T, so $230 \times 0.69 = 158$ ms. If the TI is set to 158 ms, signal from fat will be nulled. If you know the T1 time of a tissue, do the math, set the TI and suppress signal from that tissue. In Chapter 6, I referred to the null point as the transverse plane. My description showed the NMV of fat and water T1 relaxing during the sequence. Here, whatever tissues were in the X/Y or transverse plane (null point) at the end of the TI would be suppressed.

Nyquist Theorem: An important principle in digital signal processing (sampling) stating that a sine wave or signal needs to be sampled at twice its frequency to be accurate or "faithful."

Orthogonal: At 90° to another plane. Analogous to a P/A and Lateral view chest x-ray. The Lateral view is orthogonal to P/A.

Outer Lines: In k-space these edge lines contribute mostly to an image's resolution or edge detail and only a small percentage to image contrast.

Out of Phase (OOP) TE: In a GRE sequence, if the TE is such that fat and water vectors within a pixel are pointing in opposite directions, signal in that pixel will be decreased. At 1.5 T, the vectors are out of phase every 2.2 ms, so OOP at 2.2 ms, in-phase (IP) at 4.4 ms, OOP at 6.6 ms, IP at 8.8 ms.

Parallel Imaging (PI): The prime objective in parallel imaging is to image faster. The way to accomplish this is to sample fewer lines of phase. Sampling fewer phase lines comes at a price, which is SNR and resolution. There are several methods to perform parallel imaging, two of which are GRAPPA and SENSE. See "Acceleration Factor" for additional information.

Paramagnetic: If a substance has a small and positive amount of magnetic susceptibility (like gadolinium) it is considered "paramagnetic" and is weakly attracted to an external magnetic field. This quality can and will shorten the longitudinal (T1) relaxation time of a tissue. A property of Para magnetism is having unpaired electrons, which is the opposite of a diamagnetic material.

Partial Echo (also called Fractional Echo): This option is usually employed during a CE-MRA sequence. Here only about three quarters of the echo is sampled. The reason for truncating (cutting) the echo is purely to save scan time.

Partial Fourier: Related to symmetry of k-space. Slightly more than half the k-space is filled so a pattern in k-space is recognizable. The unfilled lines are filled with data discerned from the pattern in the filled lines.

Partial Volume Effect: When a tissue appears less bright or less dark than it actually should be is. When large pixels contain both bright and dark tissues, the resulting pixels will display as grey. A pixel's signal intensity is the average of all tissues inside of it. Fix: Smaller pixels and/or thinner slices.

Passive Shim: See "Hard Shim."

Perfusion: When a tissue has a blood supply you could say that it is perfused. Perfusion sequences are commonly performed in the brain during the work-up process for a stroke.

Perfusion Study: See "Dynamic Susceptibility of Contrast."

Perfusion Weighted Imaging (PWI): Another name for DSC. Basically, like any other sequence or set of images, its contrast is based on or "weighted with" the perfusion of the tissues as IV gadolinium arrives and enters the tissues.

Peripheral Nerve Stimulation (PNS): A consequence of very rapid and intense magnetic field gradient applications. It actually comes from the rapid switching or alternating polarity of the magnetic fields. This rapid switching causes small amounts of current to form and flow in the nerves of the hands and feet while the sequence is running. PNS stops when the sequence stops.

Permanent Magnet: A type of magnet made up of many magnetic bricks so that, when aligned in the right orientation, their collective magnetic fields will add up to a strength great enough to be used for imaging.

Phase: Describes the state or quality of an NMV. When all vectors/protons are pointing in the same direction they are thought to be in phase. As they spread or fan out, they are thought to be de-phasing and signal drops.

Phase Conjugate Synthesis: A mathematical premise that a number (scanned data in k-space) has an equal and opposite number value. Basically k-space is a mirror image of itself. This is the half or partial Fourier option to save time.

Phase Contrast (PC): A GRE based sequence used in MRA, MRV, CSF flow studies, and some cardiac exams.

Phase Encoding: In a pulse sequence, phase encoding happens in between excitation and refocusing. It puts each echo just a little bit more out of "phase" with the preceding echo.

Phase Encoding Gradient (PEG): A gradient applied between the 90° and the 180° RF pulses as part of spatial localization. The PEG and/or phase is sometimes symbolized as "φ".

Phase Over-Sampling: An option used to decrease or eliminate the wrap artifact or aliasing. Aliasing is seen in the phase direction. The "over-sampling" means that extra lines of phase are sampled so that the tissue that is outside the FOV in the phase direction is "sampled" enough to satisfy the Nyquist Theorem. Those extra lines are then discarded by the scanner and not displayed in the final images.

Physical Gradients: The X, Y, and Z gradients that make the classic noise during an MR sequence.

Pixel: Is a two-dimensional picture element. A pixel's dimensions result when the FOV is divided by the scan matrix. A pixel's dimensions are width × height. Pixels are the smallest visible part of a digital image.

Poor Man's Fat-Sat: A way to lower signal from fat and other background tissue simply by increasing the flip angle (F/A) in a 2D TOF MRA sequence. Increasing the F/A while using a very short TR increases the contrast between the bright vessels and a dark background, which is a desirable effect in MRA studies. Note the key term here is "in a 2D TOF MRA." The same effect in a 3D TOF comes from using a ramped pulse.

Post Labeling Delay (PLD) In Arterial Spin Labeling

(ASL): This is the time from "labeling" the spins (actually exciting the arterial blood flow) with an RF pulse to the TE. "Labeled" spins entering tissues will cause a small amount of signal loss whereas tissue that is not perfused will be slightly brighter, a non-contrast perfusion study as it were. The PLD is a user selectable value. A typical adult PLD is in the 1500–2000 ms range. As blood flow slows (i.e. in the elderly) the PLD should be increased to about 2500–3000 ms; with fast flow the PLD should be decreased to say 1000–1500 ms. These are general numbers/guidelines and are empirical. There are several factors that influence what PLD to use. These include of course age, cardiac output, the patient's hematocrit, and sickle cell anemia.

Precession: Rhythmic gyrations or spins of a body (proton) around its axis like a spinning top. The angle off of its axis is a function of a torque or pulling from an external force, that force being the magnet.

Precessional Frequency (PF): Sometimes symbolized as ω (omega). PF does not exist with the presence of B_0.

Pre-scan: At the beginning of a sequence, the scanner will adjust or tune several critical things: The center frequency of the center slice, the transmitter gain (strength), and the receiver gain.

Proton Density (PD, also termed Hydrogen Density or Spin Density): A tissue characteristic related to the number of protons in a mm^3 (cubic mm) for a given tissue (e.g. CSF vs. muscle). CSF has many more protons in a mm^3 than does muscle.

Proton Electron Dipole Interaction (PEDI): Water protons attach to the free electrons in a gadolinium molecule, letting the water release its extra energy from the RF quicker than it normally would. The T1 time of water is shortened.

Pulse Sequence Design or Line Diagram (PSD): A group of lines with symbols depicting RF and gradient applications over a time line.

Quantum Mechanics: A branch of physics centered on very small objects. The body of scientific laws describing the behavior of protons, electrons, and other sub-atomic particles.

Quench: A sudden loss of the superconductivity of the current in the magnet's coil. Loss of the cryogen causes resistance in the coil and magnetism is lost rapidly.

Radial Imaging: Often used when imaging the bile duct and gall bladder during an MRCP exam. Multiple thick slices are imaged at increasing (or decreasing angles), all having a common "pivot" point. These slices fan out like a wagon wheel.

Radiofrequency (RF): An oscillation rate of alternating electric current/voltage or electromagnetic field. The frequency range is from approximately 20 kHz (kilohertz or thousand hertz) to around 300 GHz (gigahertz or billion hertz).

Ramped Pulse: In a 3D MRA sequence, to lessen the effects of in-plane saturation, the RF pulse applied to the 3D slab has an increasing flip angle. This special kind of RF pulse increases the flip angle related to its position in the imaging slab. The idea of this higher flip angle is not to make the blood brighter, but to increase the saturation of the background tissue even further, which will increase the contrast between vessels and the background.

Rapid Acquisition with Rapid Excitation (RARE): The original term that eventually became FSE/TSE.

Raw Data: This term for the MR tech typically refers to the images generated from the TOF MRA sequence.

Real Time: See "Cine Loop."

Rectangular FOV (Rec. FOV, sometimes called Phase FOV): The FOV is square (e.g. 200 × 200 mm) unless otherwise stated, as in Rec. FOV (e.g. 150 × 200 mm). In order to save time, Rec. FOV does not scan all the lines in the phase direction as dictated by the scan matrix. Resolution is **not** affected as the scan matrix is not changed; it is just that fewer lines in the phase direction are scanned. For example, if phase is left to right in the brain, and the FOV in the phase direction includes some area without anatomy, this area (likely to be air) will not be scanned. SNR does/will decrease when using the Rec. FOV option.

Refocusing Pulse: The 180° pulse applied at half the TE and used to correct for magnetic field inhomogeneities and susceptibilities. The 180° pulse is placed "symmetrically" (halfway) between the 90° and TE.

Region of Interest (ROI): When scanning an area of suspected pathology such as a soft tissue mass within a larger area, this is called the region of interest.

Relaxation: In MRI, the act of the protons returning to a lower energy state (releasing energy) from the effects of an RF pulse. See also "T1" and "T2" relaxation.

Relaxation Curve: A graph depicting a number or volume of protons that have returned (regrown) to B_0 over time. Typically, two curves are shown in order to compare a fast-relaxing tissue to a slower-relaxing tissue. See also "Decay Curve."

Re-ordered *k*-Space Filling: In FSE or TSE where lines of *k*-space are not filled sequentially but in an order where ETE goes into center lines of *k*-space for best image contrast.

Re-phasing Gradients: These magnetic field gradients are used to re-focus or re-phase a set of vectors much like the 180° RF pulse does in a spin echo pulse sequence. These gradients are applied in an equal and opposite polarity to the previous gradient to counter its effects. They are often used in "steady state" GRE sequences. See "Re-winding Gradients."

Resistive Magnet: A type of magnet that is a large coil of wire with current flowing through. The flowing current produces a magnetic field strong enough to be used for imaging. This type of magnet also produces heat as a result of resistance in the conductor.

Restricted Diffusion: Usually used to describe an area in the brain that is involved in or an evolving CVA. When brain cells have a good blood supply, they will diffuse in a normal fashion or rate. When the blood supply is interrupted, cells begin to run out of fuel and diffusion begins to slow down/stop. This is called restricted diffusion.

Re-winding Gradients: Another name for re-phasing gradients. These magnetic field gradients are used to re-focus or re-phase a set of vectors much like the 180° RF pulse does in a spin echo pulse sequence. They are often used in "steady state" GRE sequences.

Ringing Artifact: Sometimes exchanged with the term truncation. This is an "edge" or ringing artifact that looks like alternating black and white stripes. It is caused by sharp edges of high and low signal intensities as in the bright CSF and the dark cord in the spine. It can never be completely eliminated, only lessened. The fix is to increase the scan matrix.

Rise Time: How fast a gradient can get up to a required strength. It is stated in ms and can be anywhere from 0.4 ms down to a fast 0.1 ms. Overall, rise time is useless unless coupled with slew rate.

Rupture View: View used when performing a breast study looking for a "ruptured" implant. The image contrast desired to see a ruptured implant changes with the type of implant. A saline rupture is easily seen with either a T2 fat-sat or STIR (sequence of choice is a radiologist preference). A silicone rupture view may require a STIR sequence to suppress fat, and a "water suppression" pulse which will leave only silicone to be bright on the resulting images. These two techniques are only stated as descriptions. Your department protocol should be followed.

Saddle Coil: A coil configuration in which one coil is placed on top of another surrounding the anatomy to be imaged.

Sagittal Plane: Assuming the patient is head first and supine, sagittals transect the patient from left to right. The "X" direction.

Saturation: When a tissue receives too many RF pulses over a short period of time, that tissue losses its ability to generate signal because it has little time to T1 relax. Saturation usually means that a specific tissue such as fat was targeted with RF to give little signal.

Saturation Pulse (Sat Pulse, Sat Band): An RF pulse applied either inside or outside the FOV, either for artifact control or to saturate one side of the vascular tree to null signal in blood vessels entering the slab or slice during an MRA/MRV.

Sensitivity Encoding (SENSE): A parallel imaging method where individual coils are assigned to gather specific lines of k-space. Scan time decreases in relation to the number of elements in the coil. Wrap artifact can be an issue with this method.

Sequential: In increasing (e.g. 1, 2, 3, 4) or decreasing (4, 3, 2, 1) order. Acquiring slices in said order.

Short Time (Tau) Inversion Recovery (STIR): Variation on a spin echo sequence to suppress signal from short T1 relaxing tissues, usually fat.

Signal to Noise Ratio (SNR, S/R): Simply put, the amount of signal generated in the coils over an amount of background noise. Ideally there is more signal generated by the sequence than there is background noise in the system.

Single Shot: When imaging rapidly and all the lines of phase are filled in one (1) TR period from a single 90° RF excitation pulse.

Slew Rate: A statement of gradient performance which is a combination of rise time and maximum gradient strength. It is stated as Tesla/meter/second (T/m/s). Maximum gradient strength ÷ rise time = slew rate. A good slew rate is 150–200 T/m/s; average 100–120; low fields come in at around 50–60. Slew rate affects TR, TE, and echo spacing.

Slice Excitation: An RF pulse that excites a particular region of tissue into the X/Y plane, whether it be an axial, sagittal, coronal, or somewhere in between as an oblique. It is either a 90° RF pulse in a spin echo or a partial F/A in the case of a GRE sequence.

Slice Gap: An area in between slices that is not imaged. It is usually a small percentage of the slice thickness, about 10–20%.

Slice Refocusing: An RF pulse that refocuses or re-phases a slice's X/Y plane NMV.

Slice Select Gradient (SSG): Is the gradient applied during the RF excitation to produce either an axial, sagittal, or coronal slice.

Smart Prep/Fluoro Trigger: Vendor-specificoptions/ sequences to inject a bolus of IV contrast and initiate data acquisition when the bolus reaches the target vessel.

Sodium Pump: In cellular respiration, a living cell pumps or diffuses various chemicals and waste products in and out of itself to maintain homeostasis. The sodium pump requires a blood supply to perform this task.

Spatial Resolution: The ability to see or image a structure in "space." A fancy way of saying resolution.

Specific Absorption Rate (SAR): The amount of RF energy absorbed by the patient. It is measured in watts of energy per kilogram of body weight.

Spectral Attenuation (or Adiabatic) Inversion Recovery (SPAIR): Basically, a STIR sequence with the exception being that the 180° RF pulse is tuned to the PF of fat whereas in STIR it is not. The 180° RF pulse is also repeated several times during the TR to suppress fat better.

In STIR the 180° is a wide bandwidth RF pulse that excites the entire slice. The 180° in SPAIR excites only fat.

Spectral Inversion Recovery (SPIR): A STIR sequence in which the 180° is tuned to the PF of fat and is applied only once. SPAIR and SPIR are a bit more forgiving when doing fat-sat than a true fat-sat sequence when the FOV is large and/or off-center.

Spin Angular Momentum: Protons spin on their axis like wobbling tops. Spin angular momentum comes from the proton's spin being pulled on by the magnet. The proton wants to spin upright; the magnet is trying to pull it down. The proton's "momentum" is altered.

Spin Echo: One of the two pulse sequences in MRI, the other being the GRE. Spin echo is characterized by a 90–180° RF pulse which then leads to an echo. The 90° RF pulse knocks the protons down into the X/Y plane; the 180° flips or spins them around. The resulting echo is called a "spin echo."

Spoiled Gradient Echo (SPGR): A T1 weighted GRE sequence. Vendor-specific names include BRAVO, MP-RAGE, LAVA, VIBE, VIBRANT, TRIVE, TIGRE, T1-FFE, SARGE, 3D-Fast FE, etc.

Spoiling/Spoiled: Spoiling is a method to remove residual magnetization in the transverse plane. It is done with either an RF or gradient pulse.

Spectroscopy: A sequence that is able to give a quantitative value for the concentration of metabolites. Spectroscopy is most often used in the brain to characterize brain lesions. See also "Metabolites."

Spin-Lattice: Protons heat slightly from the energy of an RF pulse. They give off this heat/energy to the surrounding tissues, known as the "lattice," in order to reach thermal equilibrium. Another name for T1 relaxation.

Spin-Spin Relaxation: When a group of protons are spinning and interacting with each other and also affecting the magnetic field between them, they will de-phase. This de-phasing from bumping into each other is called spin-spin relaxation, also known as T2.

Stagnant Flow: In a blood vessel, this is blood flowing at a very slow rate.

Static Magnetic Field: The stationary (not time-varying) main magnetic field which is the heart of the MR scanner. It is sometimes referred to as B_0. Varying magnetic fields are the gradients.

Steady State: Refers to the state of the NMV when the TR is shorter than both the T1 and T2 of a tissue. The transverse NMV stays at the F/A imparted by the RF so it neither increases nor decreases. It stays "steady."

Subtraction: A post processing function done either manually or automatically by the scanner where a "pre contrast" data set is subtracted from a "post contrast" set. The resulting set of images should be a representation of gadolinium-filled structures or tissue.

Superconducting Magnet: The most common type of magnet. It is a resistive magnet with the conductor bathed in a liquid cryogen that all but eliminates resistance in the conductor, allowing for much more current to flow and produce a stronger static magnetic field.

Suppression: A tissue or tissues are purposely made to give less signal at TE. Usually done in an IR type sequence through a combination of RF pulses and timing to allow more or less T1 relaxation. See also "Saturation."

Surface Coil: A flat RF receiver placed over or under an ROI.

Susceptibility: The idea that something can be influenced by another and to what degree. Some human tissue (e.g. fat or CSF) is susceptible to a magnetic field whereas air is not.

Susceptibility Weighting Imaging (SWI): Obtaining image contrast based on susceptibility differences between tissues. There are some vendor-specific sequences that obtain these kinds of images. These sequences are EPI and are higher resolution than most EPI sequences. If you think of it, your basic GRE (T2*) sequence, run routinely in the brain, is susceptibility weighted. You are looking for blood/hemorrhage which causes a susceptibility artifact.

Swap Phase and Frequency: There are three directions in an MR image: Slice, phase, and frequency. In swapping phase and frequency, you change their directions by 90°. This is done to "move" an artifact, make motion go in a different direction, or take advantage of a rectangular FOV and decrease scan time.

T1: Related to a relaxation rate. It is a logarithmic time constant for when 63% of a tissue has returned to (regrowing into) the longitudinal or B_0 (37% remains in the X/Y).

T2: Also related to a relaxation rate. A logarithmic time constant for when 37% of a tissue's NMV are still in the transverse or X/Y plane after the excitation pulse has been turned off (think: 63% went back to B_0).

Note: T1 and T2 are completely independent of each other but occur simultaneously. Tissues T2 and T1 at the same time.

T2*: Always associated with a GRE sequence, T2* contrast comes from inhomogeneities in the main and local magnetic field. Basically, it is the contrast you get as a result of not having a 180° pulse cleaning up for the Big Three. GRE axials in the brain are T2* and are used to look for blood.

T2 Shine Through: In DWI imaging, tissues with a very long T2 relaxation time are bright (shine through) and do not represent areas of restricted diffusion. The long T2 times can mimic stroke. The eADC is sometimes used by the radiologist as a "tie-breaker" to differentiate between a CVA or some other pathology. The eADC map removes T2 shine through from a DWI image.

Tau: Greek letter (T or τ) symbolizing time. 1 Tau= ½ the TE.

Temporal Resolution: The ability to image quickly over time. A dynamic CE-MRA is said to have high "temporal resolution."

The Big Three: Local and main magnetic field inhomogeneities, and magnetic susceptibility.

Time of Flight (TOF): An MRA concept that images with very short TRs and TEs. The TR/TE times are shorter than the T1 relaxation time of the background tissue. Background tissues quickly saturate because of the short TR/TE and with fresh **unsaturated** spins entering the slice/slab, they give off more signal than background tissue. An alternative term for time of flight is flow related enhancement.

Time of Inversion (TI): The TI is stated in ms. Long TIs suppresses long T1 relaxing tissue, short TIs suppresses short T1 relaxing tissue.

Time of Repetition (TR): The time from the 90° RF pulse that excites slice 1 to the next 90° that excites the same slice again.

Time to Echo (TE, also known as 2Tau): The time from the 90° to the 180° is 1 Tau, and from 180° to the echo is 1 Tau. 1 Tau + 1 Tau = 2 Tau. Time to echo is the time when the protons come into phase and generate signal in the coil.

Timing Bolus: In CE-MRA, filling the center lines of k-space at the same time the gadolinium bolus arrives at the target vessel is vitally important. A timing bolus sequence tells you how much time it takes for the gadolinium to get to the target vessel. See also "Smart Prep and Fluoro Trigger."

Tissue Saturation: When a tissue or tissues are exposed to RF pulses, they will want to "relax" after the RF to release the energy. If they are re-exposed to another RF pulse before sufficient relaxation has occurred, they will not be able to give off much signal at TE and are considered to be "saturated."

Torso Coil: A large receive-only surface coil used for imaging larger body parts such as the abdomen, pelvis, or long bones.

Transmit/Receive (T/R): A coil that can transmit an RF pulse as well as receive one. This kind of coil is different from coils that can only receive RF, not transmit RF.

Transmitter Bandwidth: Used in describing an RF pulse. A wide transmitter B/W contains many frequencies and will excite or refocus a wide or thick slice vs a narrow B/W which excites a thinner slice as it has fewer frequencies.

Transverse Net Magnetization Vector: The sum of vectors in the transverse plane or X/Y plane. It is at 90° to B_0. Sometimes the word "residual" is added to the beginning. This refers to how much transverse NMV is still in or left over in the X/Y plane after the TE. Its opposite or counterpart is the longitudinal NMV. This is what exists prior to excitation.

Transverse Plane (also known as the X/Y plane): It is at 90° to the longitudinal or B_0.

Truncation Artifact: Often substituted or exchanged with Gibbs artifact. It is commonly seen where there is a high degree of signal intensity differences between tissues, as on sagittal views of the cervical spine. It looks like a zebra stripe. It is caused by the signal being sampled too slowly. If we could sample the signal continuously an infinite number of times, we would not get truncation artifact.

Turbo Spin Echo (TSE): A sequence where multiple echoes are acquired per slice per TR. Synonymous with "Fast Spin Echo."

Tuning: The scanner is adjusting resonant frequency of the system components receivers and transmitters to the Larmor frequency for the optimum signal return.

Turbulent Flow: In a blood vessel, this is a flow pattern that is starting to get/go back to normal. Vectors are "pointing" all over the place. Signal from this blood is less than that from laminar flow.

Vector: A quantity of having both magnitude (amount) and a direction (Z or X/Y). Often represented by an arrow with its length proportional to its magnitude and pointing in a direction.

Velocity Encoding (Venc): A user-selectable parameter in PC imaging referring to the speed of the tissue you want to image. The venc is the maximum velocity that will be encoded into the image. Venc is increased for fast-flowing blood and decreased for slow.

Vortex Flow: In a blood vessel, a tumbling, swirling pattern of flow. It results from the blood jetting through a stenosis. Signal from blood is rather low from this flow pattern when compared to that of laminar flow.

Voxel: A 3-dimensional picture element (pixel) that has height, width, and depth or thickness: H × W × D.

Water Excitation: A sequence that has excitation and/or refocusing pulses tuned to the PF of water. Fat is not excited so gives no signal.

Water Saturation: A sequence that starts out with RFs tuned to the PF of water for saturation. See also "Fat Saturation."

Water Suppression: Usually talked about when performing spectroscopy. The precessional frequencies of the metabolites being imaged during a spectroscopy are between those of fat and water. There is more water in the brain than fat so, for a better spectroscopy, the sequence contains a "water suppression" pulse.

Weighted or Weighting: A concept of having more of one thing over another. When an image is described as T1 weighted, it means that the contrast seen is mostly due to the T1 relaxation characteristics of tissues. There is always a mixture of all three contrasts present in any image. You cannot eliminate any one contrast, just minimize it. See the weighting triangle in Chapter 3.

White Matter (WM): Is the inner layer of brain tissue made up mostly of myelinated axons. Myelin is a fatty (lipid-rich) substance surrounding nerve cells (the nervous system's "wires"). Myelin insulates the "wires" from each other.

White Matter Tractography Diffusion Tensor Imaging (DTI): A DWI sequence capable of imaging the white matter tracts in the brain. It is akin to or has a similar imaging theory to that of TOF MRA. Diffusion of white matter cells or tracts runs mostly within the cells, similar to blood flowing in a vessel. It diffuses little through the cell membrane. White matter tractography shows the location of the tracts and can be useful in surgical planning in the brain.

Wobble (Wo, or Frequency): Also symbolized as "gamma," symbol γ.

Wrap (also known as Aliasing or Fold-over): An artifact caused by tissue being outside of the FOV in the phase direction. The Nyquist Theorem was not satisfied.

X/Y Plane: Another term for the transverse plane.

Z Plane or Axis: Longitudinal or B_0.

Suggested Reading

Books

Bartalini, L., and Gerevini, A. (2018). *Artifacts and Technical Solutions in MR Diagnostic Imaging*. AITASIT Learning Project. ISBN: 9781728734927.

Brown, M.A. and Semelka, R. (1999). *MRI Basic Principles and Applications, Second Edition*. Wiley/Liss. ISBN: 0-471-33062-0.

Bushong, S.C. (2003). *Magnetic Resonance Imaging: Physical and Biological Principles, Third Edition*. Mosby. ISBN: 0-323-01485-2.

Faulkner, W. (2001). *Rad Tech's Guide to MRI: Basic Physics, Instrumentation and Quality Control*. Blackwell Science. ISBN: 0-632-04505-1.

McRobbie, D., Moore, E., Graves, M. et al. (2004). *MRI: From Proton to Picture*. Cambridge University Press. ISBN: 0-521-52319-2.

Mitchell, D. (1999). *MRI Principles*. WB Saunders. ISBN: 0-7216-6759-7.

Westbrook, C. (2008). *Handbook of MRI Technique, Third Edition*. Wiley-Blackwell. ISBN: 13: 978-1-4051-6085.

Westbrook, C., Kaut Roth, C., and Talbot, J. (2005). *MRI in Practice: Third Edition*. Blackwell Publishing. ISBN-13: 978-14051-2787-5.

Woodward, P. (2000). *MRI for Technologists, Second Edition*. McGraw-Hill Medical Publishing Division. ISBN: 0-07-135318-6.

Videos

Lipton, M. Albert Einstein College of Medicine. You-Tube MRI Physics Instructional Videos.

MRI Physics: Tech to Tech Explanations, First Edition. Stephen J. Powers.
© 2021 John Wiley & Sons Ltd. Published 2021 by John Wiley & Sons Ltd.

Index

MRI Physics: Tech to Tech Explanations, First Edition. Stephen J. Powers.
© 2021 John Wiley & Sons Ltd. Published 2021 by John Wiley & Sons Ltd.